DEADLY
DILEMMA

ANTHONY
GURLEY

DEADLY DILEMMA

A MEMOIR

MILL CITY PRESS

Mill City Press, Inc.
555 Winderley Pl, Suite 225
Maitland, FL 32751
407.339.4217
www.millcitypress.net

Due to the changing nature of the Internet, if there are any web addresses,
links, or URLs included in this manuscript, these may have been altered
and may no longer be accessible. The views and opinions shared in this
book belong solely to the author and do not necessarily reflect those of
the publisher. The publisher therefore disclaims responsibility for the
views or opinions expressed within the work.

Scripture quotations marked NIV are taken from THE HOLY BIBLE, NEW
INTERNATIONAL VERSION®, NIV® Copyright © 1973, 1978, 1984 by
International Bible Society. Used by permission of Zondervan Bible
Publishers. All rights reserved worldwide.

Lyrics from "Surely the Presence of the Lord is in This Place" are printed
with permission from Paradigm Music Productions, copyright 1977.

'To Be Or Not To Be' Soliloquy By William Shakespeare (c. 1599) -
public domain.

web address: anthonygurley.com
email: anthony@anthonygurley.com

Paperback ISBN-13: 978-1-66288-786-4
eBook ISBN-13: 978-1-6628878-7-1

Dedicated to

Maude Evelyn Worrell Gurley, who did the best she could, gave all she had and was willing to let her son pursue his dreams.

Royce Beck Smith, my father-in-law, and so much more. I could never have known when I met his daughter that I would once again have a father in my life.

Stuart Epperson, Sr. After hearing me share a brief version of this story publicly ten years ago, he told me "You need to write that down". It took a while for me to get there, but I finally did. Thank you, Stu.

ACKNOWLEDGMENTS

WHAT FOLLOWS IN this epistle is the end result of several years of remembering, reconstructing, list-making, and soul-searching. This all began as an attempt to capture Pappy's story, so my children and grandchildren might know me, for better or worse, in a way they would never otherwise know me. I owe them that much. Whatever value there is in telling this story and offering it publicly is owed to a multitude of family members, friends, schoolmates, and work colleagues.

The limits of pages and word counts would not allow me to fully express the depth of my gratitude to my high school coaches. Gerald Whisenhunt, my head football coach, led a cadre of men who reached out to me during my high school years to fill that void vacated by my absent father. Along with Coach Whisenhunt, there were Coaches Sam Shugart, Bob Waller, George Whitfield, Bill Garner, and David Odom. Hardly a day has gone by over the years that one or more of these men hasn't crossed my mind and brought back wonderful memories at times when such memories were much needed

I must also acknowledge the role Willie Frye, the pastor at Goldsboro Friends Meeting, played in my introduction to the Quaker church and all that transpired in my life springing forth from that introduction. For several years from my late teens until after I was married and started a family Willie was a role model and guiding force for me.

After high school, during my forty years at Guilford College as a student and staffer, I was blessed to come alongside many men and women who touched my life in lasting and meaningful ways. Sandy Pearman worked in my office as a work-study student when I first entered the job. Dianne Harrison, or Di, was the office secretary. Both were there for me throughout my time at Guilford. My bosses, Herb Poole, Jim Newlin, and Randy Doss, treated me with respect, always trusted my performance, and stood by me in difficult times. I can never thank them enough.

The first time I shared a synopsis of my story was before a group of Christian brothers, at the Winston-Salem chapter of the New Canaan Society. The seeds were sown that grew into a thought of capturing the story in greater length for my family and maybe a few close friends. Unexpectedly, Stuart Epperson, Sr. reached out to me afterward and told me I should "write that down". If anyone reads this rendering and is moved to deal with their struggles and challenges in a constructive way, I must say "Thank God" and his messenger, Stu Epperson, Sr.

Once I undertook the task of "writing it down", I shared the opening letter with a lady in our church and a long-time friend of the family. Lynette Hampton has been a published novelist most of her adult life under the pen name Agnes Alexander. After reading The Letter at the beginning of the story, Lynette told me I needed to rethink my plans. She encouraged me to proceed with the assumption that this project was worthy of publishing. While it is my story and my journey, there are readers who might benefit from reading my story, perhaps motivating them to face their demons and find their anchors. To Lynette I say, "Thank you". I am a better man going down the backstretch of life for listening to Lynette's advice. Through these pages, I hope I have been worthy of Lynette's confidence.

A manuscript cannot become a good book without passing through the lens of review and editing from a trusted cadre of capable Beta readers. I want to thank Kathy Adams, Chris Arline, Bud Andrews, Jeff Thigpen, Kay Pittman, Paul Coscia, Christy Chesnut, and Lynette Hampton for their time and skilled review of my work. What finally reached the publishing presses did so only due to the honest critiques of these good friends and credible critics. I am forever grateful.

Finally, I must say "Thank you" to Becky, Scot, and Courtney. I know it was not easy for them to read some of Pappy's stories. I hope some of what they read brought back pleasant memories. I know some of what they read was new to them and totally caught them by surprise. I apologize for anything they read that caused them pain or sorrow. I am grateful for the good times and known experiences that we shared during this endeavor. I can never thank God enough for putting Becky, Scot, and Courtney into my life. Thank you all for allowing me to walk with you on your journeys. Forgive me for my missteps.

CONTENTS

The Letter... I Never Sent

Dear family and friends:

It's hard to believe I am finally at this place. I have toyed with this thought for years, decades. I have talked about studying suicide as a sociology major in college. I have told friends and family that I understood how one could get to the point where suicide made sense. I've said I understood it from an academic and conceptual standpoint, but I could never do it myself. I believed what I said.

Now, I am tired. I'm tired of the daily reminders of my many failures, my under achievements. Now in my mid-seventies, I think back to my years growing up in Fairview Homes (The Project) in Goldsboro; smart as any kid at school, but constantly feeling left out, second best. I have no memories of feeling loved by family or friends. Whether or not there was actual love present is not the point. I never felt it. Maybe that was a shortcoming on my part; even that makes my point. I never thought I was good enough—at anything. I could make top grades at school, then go home to The Project, to another world.

After 73 years of waking up every day and showing one face in public while crawling into my own dark, joyless self when away from the glaring eyes of others, I am tired of the pretense. I am tired of not understanding why I can't perform better or feel happy and joyous. Sure, there are moments when I experience each of these; but these moments are fleeting and, as I get older, less frequent. I don't know what I expected life to be like. I guess I had hoped that as I got older, somehow, it would be different. Somehow, I would feel more happiness. I would feel more joy. I would feel more of a sense of accomplishment.

Now, I don't blame anyone. I certainly don't blame my wife or children. Heaven knows they have given me no reason to blame them. It would have been easier if they had. If I could only point to their misbehaviors or ill-treatment of me, I could say, "See! See how you have treated me." But that is not the case. The failure is me. I must blame myself.

For most of my life, when I would contemplate all this, I would blame others: Daddy walking out on us; Mama not trusting me; school friends smiling and interacting at school, and rarely ever being invited to events/parties. As I grew older and left home for college and work, I withdrew even more into my shell and continued to fail even more. Withdrawing from academic life at college, leading to my dismissal, I once again found myself presenting one face among my Quaker connections and work environment, but hating every minute of my solitude- knowing I was somebody different than the person others saw. The internal struggle was painful.

It has become no less painful through the years. It became even more profound when I met and married the love of my life, and we set out to raise a family. Then, while the moments of joy and happiness did come with more frequency, the old inner heartbreak of a sense of failure, of not being good enough, still found its way into my every day. I'm not sure when, but somewhere along the way, the pain became even more hurtful. I came to realize that life was never going to be any better. No matter how much I enjoyed the love of my wife and children, I was always going to be a failure, and I was always going to be disappointed and disappointing.

I am tired of both.

So- here we are.

How does this end? There are no do-overs. You don't get a mulligan. You can't change your mind after the (f)act. You'd better be sure. My faith tells me it would be an unforgivable sin. Then again, part of the whole dilemma is I'm still trying to figure out what I believe. I have wanted to believe in God and be a "Christ-follower." Much of the time, I can't feel His presence. Is that my failure? It feels that way. I hang around a group of men who refer to themselves as marketplace Christians and talk about God and their relationships with God. We hear speakers talk about the "wondrous and mysterious works of God" in their lives. I find myself being present, smiling, praying, and yet, often feeling empty and devoid of any sense of God in my life. Sometimes I am just angry. I fear I could be wrong, and there is a God who would judge me unkindly if I intentionally ended what He has created. So, what to do?

Oh, yes—I wondered when that word would find its way into this rant—FEAR! If there is any one word that encompasses my life experience, it is FEAR. I can never remember not being afraid. I have been afraid of almost everything all my life. As a child, I was horrified to be called on in class. Then, I was scared I would not be called to be on a team. I was afraid to ask girls out on dates. (I have no clue how I got up the courage to ask Becky out, much less ask her to marry me four months later). I learned from my daddy early on not to "ask for a damn thing." Today I feel like that same child. After 73 years, it still petrifies me to ask anyone for a favor - big or small. It's a never-ending cycle; I won't ask for help. So, a small problem becomes a bigger one. The bigger problem reaches critical mass, so I either have to ask for help, or the problem manifests in even more significant and troubling ways until someone else sees the problem and some remedy is forced upon the scene.

So, before a "final decision," I have decided to reflect on this intentionally. A life marked by fear and isolation, occasionally celebrated accomplishments, more frequent failures, and an overall sense of unworthiness. There have been moments of success and adulation from friends, coworkers, and family. These are memories I cherish, and yet, regrets I cannot escape.

The question becomes: Are those peaks of cherishable memories and moments of happiness and joy sufficient in number, scope, magnitude, and frequency enough to outweigh the valleys of fear, isolation, failure, and disappointments coloring the landscape of my life? And, since there is no reason to expect my remaining years to be better in any meaningful way, why not get off the treadmill? If anything, old age, with its accompanying loss of mental acuity and the onset of physical challenges, presents an even more unwelcoming horizon.

Please understand that the potential exercising of this option should not be interpreted as a failure by anyone other than me. I want my wife and children to know I love them. I know they love me. Taking this step would cause great pain in the near term. However, I hope they understand this dilemma in no way reflects negatively on them. This would merely be the logical final act of a man grown very tired of struggling to overcome his fears and failures, a man who must decide whether those cherishable memories and moments of success, happiness, and joy are sufficient in number, scope, magnitude, and frequency to provide the inner resolve to continue the daily journey.

I don't know. I just know I am so very tired...

5/5/2023

Chapter 1

SO IT BEGINS!

SO IT BEGINS! It's hard to believe I am here, attempting to relive my life on paper. I have never kept a journal or daily log of any sort. I never thought a lot about remembering the events of the day or people whose paths I crossed, and they mine. I have never given much thought there would ever be a need for me to want to recount the events of my life. It has always seemed so inconsequential. I've never felt important, certainly not so anyone would want to read anything about me, or I would want to relive any moment or memory.

Yet, here we are. It began on October 12, 1949, in Wayne County, NC. Goldsboro was a small town about fifty miles east of Raleigh. In many ways, it seems to have gotten even smaller over the years. I was born the last of five children to Jesse Leonard and Maude Evelyn (Worrell) Gurley. Both of my parents grew up in farm families. My mother was the middle child in a family of eleven. Daddy had two brothers and some half-brothers. Goldsboro was very much a town dependent on the surrounding agricultural activity in Wayne County and surrounding areas. As I grew up and, in the years afterward, it became heavily dependent, in an economic sense, on Seymour Johnson Air Force Base, which grew out of a small WWll era army base. As the roles of tobacco and cotton in the area waned over the last half of the twentieth century, the air base grew and became increasingly critical to the financial solvency of the region.

My brother, Jesse (everybody called him Buddy), was the oldest of the children. He was about 17 years older than me. I used to kid him about being old enough to be my father. Between Buddy and me were three sisters; Emma Lee (whom everybody called Sister), Joyce, and Marlene (Faye). I am about six years younger than Faye. I was so much younger than the others I have no memory of growing up with them. My first memory of Buddy was when he came home from the Korean War. I was only 4 or 5 years old then. All I remember about him in those years was Katie, his girlfriend, who would become his wife until his death in 2016.

My two older sisters, Joyce and Sister, were out of the house when I was old enough to remember anything. The one "memory" of Joyce was her breaking my leg when I was only six months old. I don't remember it, but it became the story of legend in the family. We lived in an old farmhouse in the New Hope/Saulston area in Wayne County. The house had steps made of bricks. There were loose bricks in the steps, and Joyce, carrying me in her arms, tripped and fell. We both came tumbling down, her on top of me. I have heard the story about being in the Wayne County Memorial Hospital many times, all trussed up in some traction apparatus with ropes and weights holding my little leg in place to heal. I was so small they had a tough time keeping me in bed; the weights and ropes would lift me right up off the bed.

Sister was a sickly child. My first memory of her is well after she was grown and married, eventually raising four children.

She had polio and would forever walk with a limp with feet of different sizes, requiring her to purchase two pairs of shoes each time she needed new ones.

Before I was old enough to start school, we moved from out in the country to town. Daddy had farmed some and ran a small country store. Apparently, neither provided the kind of satisfaction or financial reward to keep us in the country. Daddy got a job as a corrections officer at the Adamsville Prison Farm. We lived in a little white house on Chestnut Street, next to the railroad tracks and only a block from the train station. When I say we, I mean Mama, Daddy, Faye, and me. The others were grown, married, and starting their own families by that time. Although we now lived in town, all our relatives on both sides of the family still lived out in the country and farmed. So, while Daddy worked at the prison, Mama worked in tobacco in the summer and early fall.

I don't remember much about those first years. My first vivid memory was Hurricane Hazel in the fall of 1954. As I said, nearly all our relatives farmed. Mama would help support the family by working in tobacco (or 'backer'), as it was commonly called. I remember being at Mama's family homeplace when the "storm came up." The backer barn was a few hundred feet from the house. By this time of the year, the green backer had been pulled from its stalks (cropped) and hung in a barn to be heated and cured. Once cured, the leaves would be sorted and tied into bundles depending on their relative size and quality. These bundles would be collected into piles in large burlap sheets and made ready to take to the local warehouse for sale in Goldsboro, or perhaps Wilson or Rocky Mount. It was a process repeated all over eastern NC and elsewhere. Backer was king in those days in that part of the world.

Back to Hazel. In those days, there wasn't the kind of satellite imagery, long-range weather forecasting, and real-time telecommunications we have today. All the folks at the barn knew that day was that a storm was comin' up. I remember Mama grabbing me and, along with the rest of the folks, mostly women, dropping what they were doing and running to the cover of the big house. I don't remember a whole lot about that day. I remember folks being scared as they realized this was not an everyday thunderstorm. It was a "fall hurricane," and it was shaping up to be a big one! I remember folks curling up together in corners of the big living room of the farmhouse. The house had large, nearly floor-to-ceiling windows. Before Mama could stop me, I found my way to one of the windows to watch what was happening outside. I didn't know any better. I could see sand and dirt blowing by. I could see grass and trees bending in the air. I could hear the wind howling. I could feel the house shaking. Then, suddenly, as Mama jerked me away from the window, I could see a whole backer barn go flying by the house, followed by a giant oak tree.

I had never seen anything like it, and fortunately, I have not seen anything like it since. I don't remember how long this went on. After a while, the weather cleared. I thought it was over, and we were safe. The grownups in the house knew otherwise. While they didn't have the kind of weather forecasting we have today, they did know then we were in the middle of a severe hurricane, not just another random thundercloud. Somebody decided we should get out of the house and go to a safer place. We were in the eye of the hurricane, and it was likely to get bad again- real soon!

Before I knew what was happening, everyone was running from the house, through the yard, and across the road to an empty field. I didn't know where we were going. We were running for our dear lives. Mama held me by the hand, and we were caught up in the group. Suddenly, I tried to stop. My beanie cap had flown off my head. That little beanie was my prized possession, and I did not want to lose it. I stopped moving and tried to get away from Mama. The beanie was tumbling across the ground, and I was determined to chase it and get it back. Mama would not let go of my hand. I protested and cried, trying with all my might to get away. I did not succeed. I never saw my beanie again. I remember it to this day. Little did I appreciate the gravity of the situation then. As a proud father of two grown children and three wonderful grandchildren, I understand my mama's lion-like strength and commitment.

As it turned out, we were running to a big roadside ditch on the other side of the field. Someone determined the ditch would be a better place to ride out the rest of the storm- and so it was. No one was seriously injured, and the house remained intact, with only minor damage. That cannot be said for other buildings on the farm and parts of the county. Hazel left its mark on eastern North Carolina and me. That old home place still stands today. It has stayed in the extended family and was renovated and restored in the 2000s.

It's been a long time since Hazel. I don't know that I have thought much about life, specifically in those years before I had much self-awareness. Returning to that place and trying to relive it proved uninteresting and of little value in the context of this exercise.

While briefly reflecting on the inconsequentiality of those brief years, I am struck by how I find myself thinking about them in the context of this overall project. I have no memories of fear or self-loathing. I didn't know we were poor. I had no sense of failing in comparison to others. If I did, I surely do not remember it.

Maybe those were the "good ole days," and I was too young to realize there even was such a thing. We were not born to stay immune to the consequences of growing up and older. So, I did- grow up and older. In going back to those early years and my introduction to life and family, how I long for that immunity. But that can never be!

Chapter 2

INTO THE WORLD

IN THE FALL of 1955, a few weeks before my sixth birthday, I started school at Virginia Street Elementary School in Goldsboro. We (Mama, Daddy, Faye, and I) had moved to town. Daddy got the job working as a guard at the Adamsville Prison Farm and we lived in that small white wooden house on Chestnut Street, right next to the railroad tracks and only a block or so from the train depot. My next-door friend, Harvey Kirby, and I would play around the tracks. No, we weren't supposed to go there. When did parental instructions otherwise stop a couple of six-year-olds from being drawn to train tracks? We would find bricks and put them on the tracks to see what a passing train would do to them. Would they knock them off? Or would the bricks be crushed under the enormous wheels? It turns out it depended. It depended on exactly how and where we placed the bricks. Maybe it also had something to do with the speed of the trains. Now and then, if we could find a penny and choose not to use it on candy at the local store, we would put it on the track. I don't know how many pennies we flattened, but it was always fun.

One of the worst whippings I ever got was because of that train track. I was six years old. There was a little local grocery store about a block from the house- close enough that Mama would trust me to go there, by myself, to get milk, bread, or potatoes, that kind of stuff. Mama would always tell me to be careful, go straight to the store, and come right back. If I took too long, she would worry, and I'd be in trouble when I got home. On this day, Mama sent me to get milk. She gave me the money, told me not to lose it, and reminded me to go straight to the store and come straight back. I did just as I was told— almost. I went straight to the store and bought the milk. (Mama would also let me have a penny of the change if there was one to get a piece of candy, my favorite-crème centered caramels). I had the milk bottle in a paper sack, and I ate the caramel as I left the store. I headed home, just a block away. Then, oops— I had a problem.

While I was in the store, a train arrived. Since we were right at the train depot, trains often would stop, rather than pass through. That's what happened. A long train (I remember not being able to see the back end, and the front end, the engine, was way down on the far side of the depot). I stopped beside the tracks and waited for the train to start up again so I could get to the other side of the tracks and go home. And I waited. And I waited! And I waited for what seemed like forever. I don't know how long it was. At six years of age, it seemed like an eternity; all I could think of was how much trouble I would be in for being late getting back from the store. After waiting as long as I could, I knew I had to get home. Mama had told me to go straight to the store and straight home, so I couldn't walk towards the depot to get around the train. I had one choice – crawl under the train and DON'T break the glass milk bottle. So, that's what I did. I got down on all fours, careful not to hit the milk bottle against the rocks between the tracks, and crawled. No problem!

After clearing the train and tracks, I ran the rest of the way home, only about a half block. I ran into the house, so proud of myself. I had obeyed Mama and gone straight to and back from the store. I was late, but that wasn't my fault; and when I explained to Mama why I was late, I was sure she would not be mad. She would be proud of how I had followed her instructions. Well- that ain't exactly how it went down. Mama was furious. I don't know that I had ever seen her that mad about anything, especially me. She was a little upset it had taken so long for me to run the errand. But that was not the source of her anger. She could not believe that I had been foolish enough to crawl under a train that could have started up again at any moment. It's not like I didn't think about that possibility. I did. That's why I waited as long as I did. After a while, even at six years old, I decided to take that chance rather than continue to let my mama's anger boil as I was increasingly late in getting back home. I was scared to death to get under that train. At some point, my fear of Mama's wrath outweighed the fear of a potentially moving train.

The only other memory I have of our time on Chestnut Street was an encounter with a Venetian blind. I was only five or six years old (we moved from Chestnut Street to Fairview Homes during my first-grade year). I'm not sure what occasion prompted my encounter with the blinds. I think it may have been the Christmas season. As I recall, I volunteered to crawl behind a partially moved-out couch to plug in or unplug something. It was lights on a newly decorated Christmas tree that required plugging in, and the only available socket within reach was the one behind the couch. I remember the sofa was heavy, and Daddy didn't want to "mess with" having to move it all over the house; hence, sliding it out a little and letting the littlest one in the place get back there and put in the plug. So, I did. It was an adventure for me.

Then, suddenly, there was this blood-curdling scream as I backed out from behind the couch on all fours. At that moment, I had no idea what had happened. However, it became all too clear, all too quickly. Suddenly, I could see blood dripping from my forehead onto the floor. Mama was screaming, and Daddy was cussing. He was hollering for somebody to get a "god-damned" towel. In moments, it seemed somebody (Daddy, I imagine) had picked me up, moved me from behind the couch, and laid me on the floor. There I was, with a towel held against my forehead, bleeding profusely while Mama cried and Daddy was deciding whether I had to go to the hospital. Well, I didn't go to the hospital. I had slid my forehead along the edge of one of the blinds. I struck it at just the right angle, and it was just sharp enough that a nice inch-long gash opened above my left eyebrow. It was not deep enough to require stitches. It was bloody enough to scare the "be-Jesus" out of my Mama and Daddy.

We only stayed on Chestnut Street for a short time after I started school. I have few memories of that time. I do remember walking by myself several blocks to school. My, how times have changed. I cannot imagine letting my six-year-old walk alone to school, particularly in a neighborhood beside a train station and full of small manufacturing places. In those days, and at that time, I loved it. On the way to school, I passed a business that, to this day, I do not know what they made or did. They routinely had barrels full of scrap paper on the sidewalk and curb. It fascinated me. There would be piles of strips and slices of paper of all colors, shapes, and sizes. I loved to play in it. I would grab it by the handfuls and take as much home as possible. Mama would fuss at me for making a mess with it. I still have a fascination for such things.

Sometime in the spring of my first year in school, we moved across town to 801-A Taylor Street in Fairview Homes. I didn't know what government-subsidized housing was then. I only knew it was nicer than the white house on Chestnut Street, and I had more kids in the neighborhood to play with. However, I did have one misgiving about leaving Virginia St. School-Marsha Hagman. Marsha was my first love, my first-grade sweetheart. I still remember telling her bye. I assumed I would never see her again. At six years old, I had no concept of time and space related to interpersonal relationships. I would see her again, but not until several years later in junior high school. We became good friends and sat beside each other at graduation.

We arrived at Fairview Homes. I started attending Edgewood School. Daddy continued working at the prison farm. Mama stayed home and raised me and Faye. Life was beginning to take on many new and impactful twists and turns. I adjusted well to Edgewood School. I was always a great student and never in any trouble. I got good grades in both academics and behavior. Soon I was becoming friends with Todd Shelby, Mac Tillman, and Bert Goodwin. There were other kids my age in Fairview Homes (The Project), but these were the ones I spent the most time with. Most of the boys my age from The Project lived in "The Circle" section of the facility, and Mama would have nothing to do with that crowd. I was not allowed to go there to play. At six, seven, and eight years old, my world was Edgewood School and this small circle of friends on our block in The Project.

I think I was happy during these years. I didn't know I was a poor kid from The Project. I performed well at school. Teachers liked me. I didn't have a lot of real friends. The few I had were good friends. I don't know whether I was always shy and afraid or if that is a part of my character that was birthed and grew during this period. As I said, I think I was happy in those days.

As a family, we didn't do much together as a unit. We occasionally went to "the country" to visit aunts and uncles. Usually, that meant going to their house on a Friday or Saturday night and sitting in their living room while the grownups talked and laughed. Sometimes there would be cousins around I could play with. Often, however, it meant sitting in the corner and being quiet. On the way home, Daddy would sometimes stop at the country store to get a dollar's worth of gas (maybe 4 gallons). If he was in a good mood and had it to spare, he would get us all "hunky" ice cream bars. This was a treat I looked forward to. (For those who don't know- a hunky ice cream bar was an elongated flat chunk of vanilla ice cream on a popsicle stick, covered with a delicious frozen chocolate coating.) Sixty years later, I still can taste them. They were always a high point, worth having to sit in the corner and be quiet while the grownups visited, even if it meant listening to Daddy telling me to be careful and not drip it in the car. "Don't make a mess, boy." Usually, my sister Faye was allowed to stay behind on these visits. She was older and could stay alone or with one of her friends in the neighborhood.

My brother Buddy decided it was time to build a house. He and his wife, Katie, were ready to start a family. They had rented in town, and then out in the country. Buddy was ready to have his own home. I only remember a little about the actual building of the house. I remember when they had to clear the land on the lot Buddy had bought. It was wonderful. Daddy would take me with him as he and a handful of other men would work to remove trees and stumps. The terrain in Wayne County is flat, and the soil is a rich, loamy black texture. So, there was little earth-moving that had to be done. The trees and stumps had to go. I remember the piles of tree wood and big, black fires burning at the end of the day.

I didn't do any work. I imagine I was more in the way than anything else. I'll never forget it. When I got home, Mama was so mad. I was black from head to toe from the dirt and the smoke. I don't know who Mama was most angry with- me for getting so dirty, or Daddy for letting me get that way. Mama made me take my clothes off at the door and head straight to the bathtub. No sooner had I sat down in the tub than the water was black as could be. I had to rinse off, drain the water out of the tub, and run clean water to finish bathing in. There was no shower. What fun!!

In the fourth grade, I began to make friends outside the umbrella of The Project. By then, I was getting to know kids at school from the "outside." One of those kids was Glenn Aycock. Glenn lived a few blocks from The Project in a nice neighborhood. His daddy owned an oil distribution company, servicing gas stations and other retail vendors. Glenn's mother did not work outside the house. She had a maid who arrived on the bus two days a week. I would ride my bike to Glenn's house and play football and basketball in his yard. Glenn's yard became a gathering place for these outdoor pickup games as we grew through middle and junior high school. Glenn and I would become dear friends through high school, even though our interests, talents, and paths took us in different directions. Glenn was my first real friend outside The Project and from a markedly different social and economic station in life. I didn't initially understand that divide, and then, when I did, I experienced both envy and resentment.

Sometime in the fourth grade, I discovered the Wayne County Boys Club. (Nowadays, it is the Boys and Girls Club. In those days, it was just the Boys Club). I don't remember how or exactly when I first visited the Boys Club on Park Avenue. However it came about—I loved it. It's hard to believe now, but I was a good athlete, and the Boys Club gave me a venue to develop those skills and receive some positive nurturing in the process. I was fortunate the Boys Clubs' football and baseball fields were just across the street from the north side of The Project. I could walk two blocks and be at practice or the games.

My mama and daddy were never physically violent with me, other than an occasional spanking I richly deserved. They were never particularly mean or cruel to me. Similarly, I have no memory of them ever going out of their way to ensure I knew they loved me; or each other. Remember, I was six years younger than my closest sibling. My brother, the oldest among the siblings, was old enough to be my father. I heard more than one time I was a mistake. They never meant to have another child after Faye. I have no memory of Daddy ever telling me he loved me. Frankly, I don't remember Mama ever telling me that either, until much later in life, when I was grown up and raising a family of my own.

So, the Wayne County Boys Club, with its year-round sports and other group outings and events, became my home away from home. That is where I learned to swim and play chess and ping pong. It is where I went on my first all-day group summer camp experience – for a whole week. It is where I first experienced the "thrill of victory and the agony of defeat" in organized sports. It is where I received my first recognition for accomplishment in the form of ribbons and trophies. It is where I was befriended by grown men who genuinely wanted to help me "do well" and "do good." I was never happier than when I was at the Club or participating on a sports team emanating from the Club. This connection would last well into my junior high school years. By that time, school, sports, and other activities would assume much of the role the Boys Club had filled. Many adult male leadership figures who had been integral to the Boys Club experience were now serving some of those roles in the school setting.

Glenn Aycock and the Boys Club were not the only things of lasting importance to which I was introduced in the fourth grade. I fell in love for the second time (remember Marsha) in the fourth grade. Her name was Edie Hampshire- and I didn't have a chance. Edie was beautiful and sweet. And she stayed that way all through high school and beyond. There's an interesting story about our paths intersecting again many years after high school. More on that later! In the fourth grade, I had a real crush on Edie. For the first time, I realized I didn't measure up somehow. I was shy and afraid to speak up. And I was from The Project. You see, Glenn liked Edie too. And, although I was a much better student and athlete than Glenn, he dressed better. His mom picked him up in her car. He had money. Even in the fourth grade, those distinctions began to manifest themselves. For the first time I remember, I saw myself as second class. I could not compete- not really. That feeling would have lingering implications for the rest of my life.

After the fourth grade, I moved to William Street School for the fifth and sixth grades. I was riding a school bus for the first time until I convinced my mama to let me ride my bicycle.

After school, I could go to the Boys Club or the Community Building (basketball and swimming). I would go to one or the other places many days after school and then ride my bike home to The Project, often after dark. I cannot imagine allowing my child to do that today. The times- they have changed. These were some of the best times of my life. During this period, I met a friend who would become one of my closest friends. We don't see each other often. We talk only occasionally. Bud Andrews has had a profound impact on my life. As this story unfolds, Bud will surface time and again. Our first introduction occurred during this middle school time.

Bud tells the story about going to a Boys Club basketball championship tournament in the Community Building with his dad. I was 10 or 11 years old. I remember the event. My team was playing in the championship game. For whatever reason, our team was shorthanded. The coaches agreed to let the game go on without our having to forfeit. I don't remember much about the game, just that we fought to the bitter end and nearly won. We did lose, and I cried like a baby. I wanted so much to win, and we almost did, even though we played with only four players. Bud would later tell me that he told his dad that night that he wanted to meet that little boy crying after the game. He had never seen anybody (my words now, not his) with so much passion for the game. He thought that kid would make a good friend. We would become acquainted later, only really becoming good friends in high school.

The years at William Street School would become the transition from living primarily within the cocoon of The Project and a small circle of friends to branching out to a much broader group of acquaintances (if not friends) and wrestling with the universal challenges of growing from childhood to adulthood.

While there were great moments, to be sure, these were years when I began to think consciously about life and things that matter- and realize I was not a happy person. It was also when I began to see hints of what would result in my parents' divorce. I was ten years old at the time. It was a Saturday, and I wanted to go to the Boys Club for an evening party. I don't remember the special occasion, but there was a party at the club that night. I only got to go to that sort of thing if Glenn was going and his mom or dad, or older brother, would take us. Then, I could get a ride with him. On this evening, Daddy said he would take me and pick me up when the Club closed at 9:30. So off I went. I had a great time. When the party was over, I went outside to the street to wait for daddy. Folks were leaving the Club. Cars were stopping, picking up other kids. Finally, the crowd cleared out, and I was the only one left at the curb. The lights were off in the big colonial house that served as the home for the Boys Club. I was alone, in the dark, on the street, after 10:00 at night. I was scared. Remember, this was a time before cell phones. I had no way to call anyone. I didn't know if something had happened to Daddy. I know Mama was worried and was going to be mad. I cried. Finally, Daddy drove up around quarter past ten, forty-five minutes after the Club had closed, and way past the time I was supposed to be home. I was so relieved when I saw it was Daddy. I knew there was going to be hell to pay. I didn't know why he was so late, and he did not explain. He just told me to get in the car. When we got home to the apartment at Fairview, Mama had been crying. I was told to go to bed. I did. I don't know what was said between the two of them, but they did argue. I fell asleep before they went to bed. I don't remember whether Daddy stayed home that night or not. I didn't think much about it afterward, other than to wonder why Daddy was so late. Then, I began to notice things. Daddy was never one to talk on the telephone much. I don't remember ever seeing him on the phone. We had one telephone (wired, not wireless in those days) located on a chair/table in the short hallway between the living room and the bedrooms. I occasionally noticed that the part of the phone you lifted off the cradle and spoke into would be placed on the cradle backward. It would be in the cradle with the end from which the wire extended, opposite from the cradle's side where the wire came out. At first I didn't think anything about it. I had never seen the handpiece lying there backward before. Nobody put it back down like that. I then began seeing ashes in the ashtray on the table also. Daddy was the only one in the house who smoked. Mama dipped powdered tobacco (snuff). Soon, I put it together that Daddy was talking on the phone when nobody else was in the apartment.

About this time, something else began to occur. As I noted earlier, our apartment in The Project was about a block and a half from the city-owned sports complex where the Boys Club played football and baseball games. The property also contained several softball fields where the adult softball leagues played. Some nights Daddy would take me to watch these games. I didn't care much for the softball games. It was one of the few times we spent any time together. So, off we would go. I remember almost having to run to keep up with Daddy's big steps as we crossed the open field leading to the softball fields and parking lots. Once we got to the games, Daddy would let me roam free.

I felt so grown up. There were usually at least one or two kids there I knew from The Project. At the time, I didn't pay attention to the time or where Daddy was. I knew I was supposed to be at a certain spot when the games were over. Daddy and I would walk home then, getting away from the fields before they turned out all the lights. I don't know when I first noticed it. One such night the games were over, and I was at my spot, but not Daddy. I began to be afraid, wondering if something had happened to him. I began to wonder if I should walk home without him. You could see the block of apartments where we lived from where I was waiting. They were just across the field and down the block. Finally, he arrived, out of breath and mad about something. He said he had been looking for me and couldn't find me. I had been right where I was supposed to be. I knew better than not to be there. I had felt the sting of Daddy's belt enough times to know better than to invite it intentionally. That sort of disconnect at the games would occur now and then. I never got a whipping for it.

At first, I didn't put it together. Much later, after he left, I found out he was seeing another woman who lived around the corner and down the block from our apartment. Louise Adams was a divorcee with a daughter in the same grade as me. I knew her from school, although we were not friends. Later, after Daddy moved out, he moved in just around the corner. I remember occasionally seeing him in the backyard of her apartment, walking behind one of those old walk-behind reel mowers, mowing her yard. Even then, I thought it strange. I had never seen him mow our small yard. That was always my job.

Alas, I am getting ahead of myself. Although these things percolated in the background during this period, I was growing up independent of it all. My life revolved around school and sports, and I excelled at both. My teachers loved me and encouraged me. I read all the time. I loved biographies and histories. I remember reading about George Washington Carver and being fascinated by his accomplishments. I was in the fifth grade at the time. When folks did their laundry, they ironed almost everything back in those days. One of my jobs was to help Mama with the wash. She had a "portable" electric washing machine. It was a big tub with a wringer attachment at the top. Mama would roll it from the pantry closet to the kitchen sink. It had what looked like a short garden hose and drain hose. She would fill the tub with water from the kitchen sink, put in the detergent, plug it in and turn on the switch. The machine would begin agitating the clothes she had loaded. After washing them, Mama would drain the water into the sink. Then she would commence several cycles of running the clothes through the top-mounted wringer, a device consisting of two rolling pins, connecting with a hand-turned crank on one end. As you fed the clothes, one or two pieces at a time, the turning crank would draw them between the two rolling pins and squeeze water from them. After all the clothes had gone through this process, Mama would run them through again, extracting even more water. When she was satisfied she had gotten all the water the wringer would get out, she would drain the tub, wipe it with a rag to dry it, and return the machine to the pantry. Some items had to be starched. Mama would put them in a water bowl into which she added starch. She would then take all the wash, starched and unstarched, to the clothesline in the back-yard to dry in the sun, hanging them with wooden clothes pins. After the clothes were dry, Mama would bring them in. Often I would help, sometimes doing the entire gathering all by myself. The unstarched items were either folded and put away, or ironed before being put away. The starched items had one more step before being ironed. Mama would put water in a tall Pepsi Cola bottle with a stopper with holes in the top. She would sprinkle the starched items, roll them up neatly, put them in a plastic bag, and place them in the refrigerator until she was ready to iron them. This is where George Washington Carver comes in. Mama taught me how to iron, which became a regular chore. I became pretty good at it, a talent my wife, many years later, would appreciate. I did not enjoy it, and sometimes I hated my mama for making me do it. And then I read George Washington Carver's biography. He wrote about helping his mama as she did laundry for other folks. She taught him to iron and help her when the load was just too much for her to do it all by herself. It came upon me as an epiphany. Who was I to balk at doing it if he could do it? I was amazed at all he had accomplished, doing so in his era. It never occurred to me how unusual it might be for a poor white kid from The Projects in a small town in eastern North Carolina in the 1950s to develop such an appreciation and respect for a Black crop scientist. To this day, I do love good creamy smooth peanut butter and honey-roasted goobers!

Looking back at these six years or so, I am struck by how different times are today. It was a pivotal time, from playing on railroad tracks with a next-door neighbor to walking to school and spending half my waking hours outside the confines of my home. Everyone didn't go to daycare, preschool, or kindergarten in those days. Some did, and many didn't. Certainly, kids who lived next to the tracks or in The Project didn't. Entering public school introduced me to a new cultural class, particularly after transferring to Edgewood

School. There I encountered a more diverse socio-economic culture (I had no idea that term even existed then. It did not include a racial component. That would come later in the tobacco fields.) I do have memories of those years. I remember being afraid. For the first time in my life, I experienced envy and embarrassment. I was poor and was beginning to have some understanding of what that meant. It was much later in life that I consciously understood it was during these years that I noticed the absence of any visual demonstrations of love from my parents towards me or each other. I wouldn't experience the full result of that for a while yet.

I don't know what psychologists have to say about how and when certain developmental stages should occur in life. When does one begin to experience and understand the concepts of happiness, joy, and self-value? When do feelings of envy, anger associated with feelings, and senses of failure and disappointment begin to manifest themselves? I don't know. I'm sure I started moving down those roads during these early years with exposure to life outside The Project, only to return to 801-A Taylor Street. Perhaps this developmental picture is quite the norm, and I have let myself make way too much of it. Maybe. That does not make it any less real. It does not mean the consequences of those experiences and choices and resulting feelings are any less meaningful or causative in relation to a multitude of life's subsequent behaviors.

Chapter 3

SPORTS AS ESCAPE

IN THE 1950S and 60s, at least in Goldsboro, organized team sports began when you were nine. As soon as I was old enough, I joined the Boys Club to be able to play organized sports (and to win free passes to the Community Building swimming pool in the summer). In my first year of eligibility, I tried out for Little League baseball and made the team. I became a Civitan. Local civic clubs sponsored all six teams in the league. We had the Civitans, Lions, Elks, Rotary, Jaycees, and Kiwanis. At our first team practice, I volunteered to be the catcher.

No one else wanted to do it. I had never done it. I had no idea how to be a catcher. I did become one, though- and a rather good one at that. I would make the Little League all-star team each year I was in Little League (age 9-12). I was also a good hitter, usually batting either 3rd, 4th, or 5th in the lineup. I only hit two home runs in my entire Little League career. I consistently hit for a high average. I didn't strike out much.

I lived for Little League baseball in the spring and first half of the summer. We played two nights each week of the season. We practiced every Saturday. When we didn't have official team practice, you could always get up a sandlot game. I had no idea in those days how beautiful life was for me. I loved to play. I loved winning. Sometimes I cried when we lost. I would win trophies for achievement and good sportsmanship. In all those years of Little League, and later Junior League (ages 13-15), I don't remember either of my parents coming to see me play.

I made great friends in Little League. There were father figures introduced into my life then that I didn't begin to appreciate as such at the time. Daddy was still at home, but we never had much of a father-son relationship. There were coaches and Boys Club volunteers who filled that void. Speaking of friends, two of my Civitan teammates were Fred Arnold and Pat Richardson. Fred lived in The Project, also. Pat didn't. Fred was a good baseball player and one of the funniest people I have ever known. Pat was a short left-handed pitcher. He wasn't much of a baseball player otherwise. He grew up to be an excellent golfer, playing at the collegiate level and working as a club pro as an adult. He couldn't throw the ball very hard at all. Often, when he was pitching and we were not doing well, I would find myself firing the ball back to him much harder than his pitches were coming to the plate. We got along well, and I would go over to his house occasionally to play along with other boys from the team. I don't know what Pat's father did for a living. Whatever he did, he must have been good at it. At the time, I didn't know what rich was, but I thought they were rich. And Pat had a pretty sister. Even at that early age, I recognized pretty girls and, in my quiet and shy way, enjoyed being around them, but not too close.

One of my first travel experiences was due to Pat and his father. I was eleven years old and had never been anywhere outside of Wayne County unless it was to visit one of my parents' relatives in Green County. Pat Richardson was accustomed to going places with his family. In the summer of 1960, after my sixth-grade school year, Pat and his dad opened a door for me that I would cherish forever. Pat had been to Major League baseball games many times with his dad. This particular year Pat's dad told him he could invite two of his teammates to go with them to see the New York Yankees play the Washington Senators in a Saturday double-header in Washington, D.C. Pat asked me and Fred. Pat and his dad knew Fred and I lived in The Project and assumed we had never done anything like that before. They were right. When Pat asked me if I wanted to go, I thought my heart would explode. I had never been so excited about anything in my young life. And now, at 73, I must admit I can't recall experiencing that chest-pounding excitement and sense of deep-down anticipation very often. It would be my first professional baseball game, my first train ride, and my first time eating in a nice restaurant.

The four of us caught the train in Goldsboro for an overnight train ride to Washington. We slept in sleeper compartments on the train. I'm telling you. I could not believe it was real. Mr. Arnold knew people and had connections. When we got to the Senators stadium, before the first game, he arranged to take us into the umpires' dressing room and introduce us. We each received an official game ball. He introduced us to Pee Wee Reese, a former Yankee shortstop and future Hall of Famer. He autographed the balls we had just gotten from the umpires. I don't remember who we saw play for the Senators. On the Yankees team, we saw Whitey Ford pitch one of the games. Yogi Berra, Tom Tresh, Bobby Richardson, and Tony Kubeck were there. We saw Roger Maris and Mickey Mantle. I was in heaven. Our seats were in the front row along the third base line, just beyond the dugout. Pat caught a foul ball. I can't remember who won the games or what the scores were. I remember having the time of my life. Then I came home to The Project, and life at home was the same. I still had sports. Life at home was chores, staying out of the way, being quiet, and staying out of trouble. Don't get in front of the television and block Daddy's view. More than once, I heard, "Get out of the way. I can't see through muddy water."

The seasons changed, and so did my sports participation. From baseball in the spring and summer, I went to football in the fall and basketball in the winter- all through the Boys Club. Baseball was my favorite sport. But I was surprisingly good at youth football and basketball. In football, I played quarterback on offense and linebacker on defense. I made the all-star team. I was a guard in basketball- not tall enough to be a forward or center. I mentioned Glenn Aycock earlier. Glenn's house became the place where pickup football and basketball games took place. I spent many Saturday mornings and afternoons in Glenn's backyard with him and several other non-Project friends playing football and basketball. Oh, what I would give to relive those times.

After Little League and middle school, I moved on to Junior High School. I was eleven years old when I started junior high school. I had no idea how my life was about to change.

In the fall of 1961, I started junior high school. In those days, we had primary schools (grades 1-4), middle school (grades 5-6), junior high school (grades 7-9), and high school (grades 10-12). I was excited to make that step up. I would no longer play football (I was way too small by then). I tried out for the seventh & eighth-grade basketball team. Even though there would only be two or three 7th graders on the team, I was sure I could be one of those. I had played enough Boys Club basketball to know I was as good as the other guys who were trying out, particularly the smaller ones who would be trying out for a guard position. Basketball season rolled around, and Mama and Daddy said I could try out. I don't know whether either of them knew much about what that meant- or cared, for that matter. All I knew was that I was going to do it, and I would be a part of something special.

Tryouts began, and it was hard work. I had played sports since Little League but had never really worked at it- running drills, exercising, running coordinated plays. I don't remember how many of us there were trying out. All I remember was that I was doing well. The Coach was whittling the number down to get to his final team. Only four seventh graders left after a couple of days of tryouts. Glenn and I were still there. We were lined up at the end of the court, taking turns catching the ball and dribbling down the court to shoot a layup at the other end. The Coach was at mid-court on the far side from where we were. I was having a great time.

Those days were when Chubby Checker and "The Twist" were the rage in pop music and dance. Even at 12 years old (most of my classmates were already 13), we noticed girls in a new way, and music and dancing were becoming a part of our world. While waiting in line for our turn to catch and dribble, Glenn and I started "dancing," not really dancing, just kind of "twisting" in place. Suddenly, I heard a loud, shrill whistle. We stopped. Everybody stopped. Coach called me over to where he was sitting on the edge of the stage in the gymnatorium. (It didn't occur to me then that he only called me, not Glenn). At any rate, Coach was not happy. He told me I was cut. I would not make the team. It was because I had been clowning around when I should have been paying attention. He needed guys who could play well, pay attention, and be coached. I pled and begged for another chance. I assured him, to the extent a 12-year-old could assure a towering authority figure, that I had learned my lesson and would not make that mistake again.

I pled to no avail. I was the next to the last player cut that year. Glenn was cut the next day. I don't know whether I would have made the team or not. I believed then and still think I could have made it had I not been caught being stupid. (That would not be the last time I would suffer the consequences of "being stupid.")

I don't remember what day or date all that occurred. It was a little after my 12th birthday. I was born on October 12, 1949. I started school when I was five, turning six in October of my first-grade year. I did so without having attended any preschool or kindergarten. I was always one of the youngest in my classes. I didn't think much about it then. It wasn't until high school that I began to think about how those years impacted my social and athletic development, constantly engaging with and competing with kids as much as a year older than me.

At any rate, I was cut. I walked to the dressing room. I didn't even take a shower. I changed clothes and headed out the door to return to The Project. Goldsboro Junior High School was just a block from Goldsboro Senior High School, and both were about a mile and a half from The Project. I usually rode the school bus. When tryouts started, I convinced mama to let me ride my bicycle because I couldn't catch the school bus home after school. So, on that day, I had my bike at school. After changing clothes, I shuffled out to my bike, put my second-hand gym bag in the basket, and pedaled home, crying so hard I could hardly see the street before me. It was already dark when I left the gymnatorium. I had no light on my bike. I arrived home safely, not knowing what I was about to walk into.

So many years have gone by. My youngest grandchild is nearly as old as me in the abovementioned years. And yet, the memories are as vivid as if they happened yesterday— both the good and the bad. I can still "feel" the jostling of the train ride to D.C. I can feel the sensation of climbing into my bed on the moving train. I was in another world— going to bed on a moving train. How could that even be possible? I can also shut my eyes and hear the Coach's whistle. I can still feel my heart throb as I ran over to him, sitting on the stage steps at midcourt. I knew he would tell me I was on the team. Then, suddenly, my world came crashing down. At that age, everything is magnified in its importance. Every emotion is packed with the power to raise up or to destroy. It doesn't matter whether the reality is temporary or life-long permanent. In that moment, it is reality, and nothing can change it.

Theoretically, I guess, as we age, our experience of these emotional moments is supposed to be more manageable. I think our life experiences and normal physical and emotional maturity is supposed to equip us to manage these moments better. We are taught to learn from them. We are taught not to get too high or too low during these moments. I suppose that is true and sound advice. However, I also know the train ride to D.C. and subsequent baseball weekend is as

29

real in my emotional being as if it just happened. I don't ever want not to feel it.

On the other hand, I wish I could remember being cut from the team tryouts and why I was cut, and that be it– just a memory. It will never be "just a memory." It will always be a visceral experience every time it crosses my mind.

So, there's the good and the bad– a peak and a valley. Life is forever an unfolding saga of both. I am perplexed. I wish I could forget and never again feel the disappointment and failure of that night in the junior high gym. Sometimes, when in the throes of reliving those moments, I would give anything to never live that moment again. Life isn't like that– at least not for me. One cannot pick and choose which memories, which life experiences, and which emotionally high or low moments one must relive. That reality, at least for me, can be very taxing, very tiring!

Chapter 4

AWAKENINGS OF LONELINESS

I DON'T KNOW when I began to realize I was lonely or why I was lonely. I do know that, from a young age, I was afraid of almost everything. I didn't connect that fear with being lonely. Like most kids in those early years, I got up in the morning, living the day, never giving much thought to what could have been, or what might have been, or what should have been—until life happened and, suddenly, I was face-to-face with failure and disappointment.

When I turned the corner on my bike and arrived at the apartment, I was still crying after being cut from the tryouts. That was all that was on my mind. Life could not get any worse. Well- sometimes it can. I put down the kickstand on my bike, grabbed my bag, and started towards the screen door. Before I could get to the door, it opened- suddenly. I met Daddy walking out with a suitcase and a pile of clothes slung over his shoulder. He didn't say a word. We just passed on the walk. He stormed to his car, threw the suitcase and clothes in the trunk, and sped away. I did not know I would never see that car parked at our apartment again. Life had already taken one unexpected turn, and now another. These were turns for which that little boy in The Project was ill-prepared. I was about to launch into a journey I did not see coming. As the days passed, I began to recall the phone cord and ashes in the hall ashtray. I remembered those walks to the softball fields when Daddy "disappeared." I relived the fear of sitting at the curb of the Boys Club, waiting for Daddy to pick me up. It all began to make sense.

As I recall, I saw Daddy personally two times between that night and many years later when my children were born. On two occasions in the weeks following his departure, he waited to intercept me on my way to school. He parked near a small shopping area next to The Project. He hailed me as I walked by and offered me a ride. He could put my bike in the trunk. I was afraid. I was afraid of what mama would do if she found out. I did not ride with him on either occasion. These were brief exchanges, and we went our separate ways. After two failed attempts, I didn't see him again until years later, when my son, Scot, was born. No, that's not true. I did see him occasionally when he mowed Louise's yard. That was a couple of hundred yards away, and we had no interaction.

Junior High School, those early teen years, was a mixed bag. What began with the emotional devastation of walking into my home as my daddy walked out would evolve three years later into a place where I lived two lives. I was, at once, a smart student leader (loved by teachers). At the same time, I was also a disappointed kid who was beginning to see his athletic aspirations disappear and his "place" in the social order begin to become apparent. Those years from 1960-63 (11 to 14 years old) were typical pre-teen and early teen years in many ways-emerging hormones, changing physical and emotional behavior, and an evolving definition of the social norm in which my life was to develop. All kids go through these years and experience this cacophony of physical, emotional, and structural changes in their lives. In my case, I began to feel as though I was living two lives- one emerged when I crossed the steps to the "schoolhouse" each morning, Monday-Friday, and one took charge when I left school for the bike ride back home and every weekend day. For the first time in my life, I began to consciously experience feeling lonely. I don't think I thought about it in those terms then; that probably didn't occur until later in high school and then more so in college. In retrospect, feeling alone and lonely and feeling sorry for myself was my life then. I did not understand how that daily percolating cancer would mold my development during my teenage years and set the basis for the rest of my life. Sitting here, writing this, in my home office (my son's old bedroom in this 115-year-old farmhouse that my wife's grandfather built), I am suddenly struck by the thought of how I managed to be so successful in my work career- up to a point. Even now, I can see the same "two lives" experience previously noted in that thought vision.

During those years, I was channeled into a handful of new and different paths and social connections. Until then, my life had revolved mostly around family and The Project, with some considerable influence from the Boys Club. There had never been much expression of love for one another at home. There was also no visible expression of affection. I have no memory of ever seeing Mama and Daddy embrace one another. I don't ever remember being hugged or kissed by either of them. There was also no physical violence or alcohol or substance abuse. My playmates mostly came from The Project. Glenn was one of my few friends from outside The Project. He was the only friend I had outside The Project whose house I had ever been to and whose parents I knew. Until Jr. High school, I had attended school in the neighborhood within easy walking distance from home. With the advancement to Jr. High, I found myself in a school setting where I saw fresh faces beside old friends.

Until Jr. High, my life outside The Project consisted of occasional family visits to relatives out in the country, going with Mama to work in tobacco on relatives' farms, and sports organized by the Boys Club. I played on football and baseball fields next to The Project property or downtown Goldsboro at the Boys Club building or the Goldsboro Community Center. My geographical world was changing, getting a little bigger. My social network was expanding and evolving as well. I didn't understand the concept of sociological evolution at the time. That is what it was. Still, a pattern was beginning to form.

On the one hand, I now see a little boy being forced to mature into a big boy and then a young man, and doing so along at least two paths. One path was that of a smart student, with outward appeal as a student leader, and adapting interest in sports and how my involvement in sports could be manifested. On the other hand, I see that same little boy pretending to be that student leader and achiever; but underneath, a desperately shy child scared of failure and rejection. At school, I would see kids I wanted to be like and liked by. Then, in the quiet of riding my bike home, being at home with Mama (and later Papa), and being alone, I would go to that place I grew to know only too well. I felt sorry for myself- for what I didn't have, who I wasn't, where I didn't get to go, what I didn't get to do.

These three years were filled with what I now know are the usual rites of passage for boys (and girls) at that age. With all the personal introspection I have been citing came a new awareness of local and global happenings. From the time I was in elementary school, I was a newspaper reader, and not just the sports pages. I remember reading occasional articles in the Goldsboro

News-Argus about a war evolving on the other side of the world in a place called Vietnam. It was somewhere near China. The fighting was mainly between the people of Vietnam and a French colonial presence. The Chinese were helping the Vietnamese. Occasionally these articles mentioned guerilla fighters. I was stunned. How could they train gorillas to fight for them? I must have read dozens of such articles before discovering that the guerilla fighters were not gorillas. I was embarrassed when I realized the difference. I don't recall telling anybody about my amazement at the use of guerillas. I certainly hope I didn't.

Somewhere during this time, in my early Jr. High years, I read something about Princeton University in the newspaper. I had read enough to know that Princeton University was famous, prestigious, and one of the finest in the country. I couldn't understand how such a highly regarded, elite university could have been built in Princeton, NC. Princeton, NC, was a small hamlet (less than 1500 people today) in eastern North Carolina, less than fifteen miles from where I lived in Goldsboro. I was aware of the town of Princeton. I don't think I had ever been there. That would change once I got to high school and traveled with sports teams. At any rate, it was when I got to high school that I discovered my mistake. By then, I realized I might get to go to college somewhere. I didn't know why, other than I could get a good job if I went to college. I also learned Princeton University was a little farther from Goldsboro than Princeton, NC, and it had nothing to do with the hamlet down the highway.

In 1961 John Kennedy was inaugurated as the 35th president of the United States. In the seventh grade, I began to be aware of things beyond The Project and my little piece of it. I heard about the Peace Corps and thought early on I might like to do that. I could see some of the world and do something good for folks. I would leave The Project. About the time of my 13th birthday, our country and the Soviet Union came to the brink of a nuclear holocaust over the presence of Soviet nuclear missiles in Cuba. After days of behind-the-scenes negotiations and on the seas near naval confrontations, the two countries settled the issue, and the missiles were removed. (The US also agreed to remove some missiles from foreign stations bordering the Soviet Union.) This was not before we, as students at school, were trained and drilled on how to find refuge in school building hallways if a bomb attack occurred. Goldsboro was/is the home of Seymour Johnson Air Force Base. At that time, it was the home of the B-52 long-range bombers. These bombers were equipped to deliver nuclear bombs to the Soviet Union. We would have been a top priority target for Soviet missiles during a war. During this time, I developed a keen interest in politics and global affairs, an interest I continue to this day. I began to sense I was moving in a direction away from and apart from my family, my tradition. My interests and curiosity were beginning to be pricked. Later, in high school, a coach would open the door to further this evolution of the kid from The Project.

Previously I wrote about being cut from tryouts for the Jr High 7th & 8th Grade basketball team. I was the next to the last player cut. My friend, Glenn, was the last player cut. He and I continued our friendship. When we got to high school, he would give me a ride to school in his brand-new Pontiac GTO. I was so envious. While still in junior high, we often played basketball in his backyard. We played a lot of tennis at Herman Park. The park was only about a mile from Glenn's house and about five blocks further from my apartment. It was right across the street from the high school, where we would graduate in 1967. I would ride my bike to his house and bike together to the park. The park had all kinds of swings, slides, and playground equipment, complete with a miniature train run by the Goldsboro Kiwanis Club. In addition, it had about a dozen good, fenced tennis courts. There was also a paved practice cinder block wall. Glenn and I spent many summer and weekend hours playing tennis on those courts. Some of my few and fondest memories of these years were made on these courts. Glenn and I were pretty even in our skill level. We were different in our demeanor. When Glenn was winning, all was well. When I was getting the best of him, all Hell could break loose! He would lose control. He would cuss and throw his racket at the net or the back fence. I have seen him hit balls "miles" over the fence, cursing all the while. I didn't like losing either, but I rarely went off like that.

Nevertheless, we remained friends and continued to play. When the time came to take a break, we would ride our bikes about three blocks to Ash Street Drug Store, or Ash Cash, as the locals called it. Ash Cash was what we might today call a traditional soda shop. It had all the necessary drugstore and pharmacy items. It also had ice cream and various soda offerings. My favorite was a large cherry coke. Glenn always got a big orange-aid. I never had a lot of money then (I was too young to work in a real job, but I could save what little I earned from working in tobacco). Glenn and I would get our drinks and eat much of the ice in them before leaving Ash Cash. The drugstore was across the street from the old Wayne Memorial Hospital. I don't remember how this came about; perhaps one of our friends discovered it and told us about it. We found an unlocked door to a small room on the ground level of the west side entrance to the hospital. Therein was a huge ice machine. Glenn and I would sneak in and refill our cups with fresh ice. We would drink them all the way back to the tennis courts. Sometimes we would decide we were done for the day and enjoy the drinks all the way home.

These were some of the best times of my life. While engaged in those hours, I was as good as anybody else. I didn't have to pretend or be afraid of anything. Soon enough, though, I would be back to The Project, and the real world would return. As those years unfolded, Glenn and I did slowly inch apart. Glenn was not a particularly strong student. He struggled to pass his classwork. He was not involved in extracurricular activities at school. He was even more shy than I was. From when I started being involved with school sports programs after school to when we graduated in 1967, Glenn often got to my apartment for help with his homework before I got home from practice. As our interests at school and outside of school went their separate ways, we saw less and less of each other. By the time we were in high school, Glenn had a nice car, and I had none. So, Saturday nights would often find us together, bowling or occasionally double dating. To this day, I am grateful for our friendship. After we graduated and I went off to college, we had little contact with each other. Glenn joined the National Guard and then went to work in various jobs in Goldsboro. Glenn was a good friend.

After my daddy left, there was to be another personnel change in the Gurley household. Papa came to live with us that same year. Papa was my grandfather, my mama's daddy. Papa was old and, I would say, senile. He was bedridden and required constant care. He was the only grandparent I ever knew. He was a thin man, in his early eighties, with beautiful white hair. Until he came to live with us, he had been shuffled around among several of his children's homes. My mama was one of thirteen children, ten girls, and three boys. Age-wise, she was right in the middle of that crew. None of my aunts or uncles liked the responsibility of caring for Papa.

With my daddy out of the house and my older sister now graduated and away at business school in Raleigh, having Papa come to stay with us permanently made some sense to the family. It proved to be a real burden for Mama. Papa's physical care was demanding. He had to be fed and bathed in bed. More than the physical demands, though, was the emotional impact. Papa was not a nice person. He didn't talk much, but he was nasty when he did talk. He showed no love for Mama or appreciation for what she was doing for him. Mama was housebound for years, from when he came to stay with us to the time of his death, some six or seven years later. She could not leave just anytime to run errands, attend church, or see friends. She would get out once a month to go grocery shopping and to get a breath of fresh air. I'm sure I didn't appreciate her sacrifice during those years. I know I hated having to help him. I hated it when he would mess in his bed and scatter it, or when I had to help bathe him. I am not proud of my thoughts then. I did help Mama and never complained so she could see it.

The junior high years were filled with firsts. That's not unusual or unique to me. It feels different for all pre-teen and early teenage boys and girls. That bifurcated life I've spoken of earlier was a constant. Life, during those years, began what was to become a lifelong journey (struggle). I was constantly living in one place at one moment and then off to another realm for some unknown short period. I'll always remember my introduction to eating in restaurants and traveling outside a handful of miles from home.

After not making the basketball team as a seventh grader, I did make it the following year, and then again a year later in the 9th grade. I loved playing basketball. I loved all three major sports. Although I made the teams, I only got a little playing time. I was one of those guys who came in at the end of games when we were either way ahead or getting badly beaten. I would like to have played more. I needed to be taller, faster, and stronger. But I was on the team. That meant I spent time with coaches and guys I otherwise would not have spent much time with. I was also going to places I had never been. We would play teams across eastern North Carolina- Kinston, Greenville, Wilson, Rocky Mount, Wilmington, Fayetteville, Raleigh, and Durham. I had never been to any of these places. Sometimes we would take box meals when we traveled to play these road games. Sometimes we would eat at a restaurant, usually one of the fine eastern North Carolina Bar-B-Q establishments. I had never been inside a restaurant before I started going with school teams.

I found a way to expand this team participation beyond basketball. In the spring of my seventh-grade year, after I had failed to make the basketball team the previous fall, I managed to get a job (unpaid) with the baseball team as a manager. I wanted to play on the baseball team, but it was clear I would never play any. All through Little League, there was one catcher better than me. He would be the guy. The team needed a manager, and I wasn't too proud to do that job. The coach was the same coach who had cut me from the basketball tryouts earlier that year. The next year in the eighth grade, I would also be a manager for the junior high football team. So, by the eighth grade,

I was involved in sports throughout the school year- manager for football and baseball and sitting on the bench for basketball. Most of the year, when I left for school in the morning, I would get home again at supper or later. That was OK with me.

I did not think about my mama's effort to allow me to do this. I continued this after-school sports involvement through high school. In high school, I added the role of Head Manager and athletic trainer. That meant even longer hours. It wasn't until I was in college that I began to appreciate how much Mama sacrificed to allow me to do these things. I knew she was proud of me for what I was doing, both with sports and other school achievements. She never told me I had to quit any of this involvement and get a job after school. I knew we didn't have any money. She did receive some support for looking after Papa. I don't know how much support Daddy was required to send. But she never made me stop. She understood how important school was for me and the importance of having these coaches in my life. Mama never went beyond the eighth grade and never had a driver's license. She had never eaten in a restaurant besides a little country store diner owned by one of her sisters and a small lunch counter on Center Street in downtown Goldsboro. To this day, I am grateful for her allowing me to pursue that involvement in junior high and high school. I never adequately thanked her for her farsightedness in this regard.

Two other first-time events made a marked impression on me during these years. I have always been timid. I was poor. I was skinny with auburn (some would say red) hair and freckles. I never dated a lot during high school and never had a serious girlfriend. There were occasional after-game sock-hops, with plenty of chaperones. I would go. There usually would be a line of boys on one side of the gym and a line of girls on the other.

During the 1960s, that's how junior high school went. However, there was a group of kids "from the other side of the tracks" that was exposed to other such social engagements.

I was invited to attend a dance at the Goldsboro Country Club in the eighth grade. The girl who asked me was ridiculously cute and one of the "in crowd." We were friends at school as we shared classes. She was a cheerleader. I had never been invited to a dance and certainly not at the country club. I was terrified. My sister, Marlene (Faye), and her boyfriend took us. I was shy and embarrassed from the start. I had a suit, but it wasn't up to snuff with what the boys wore. When we arrived at the girl's house to pick her up, I was clearly not in Kansas anymore. I didn't know how to act when we arrived at the country club. I really couldn't dance much. I've always been quiet and not much of a small talker. I couldn't believe I was where I was and with one of the cutest and most popular girls in school. I didn't want the night ever to end —and I couldn't wait for it to be over. That night was sixty years ago, and I still remember how I felt. At once, I was where any boy in school would have dreamed of being, and with a girl I could only dream would "like" me. At the same time, I felt so out of place, as uncomfortable as I had ever felt or have ever felt since.

As elevated as I was that night and as uncomfortable as I was, I willingly encountered the same situation again in high school. Another beautiful girl, a well-liked student leader, and a cheerleader, invited me to another Country Club Dance. We were acquaintances in high school but traveled in vastly different circles. You can imagine my surprise when she asked me to a dance at the Club. This was during our junior year. I guess the visceral impact of my junior high experience had subsided by then. I said yes and looked forward to the date. The evening unfolded a lot like the earlier experience in junior high school. When my date invited me to the event, I didn't know where she lived. When she gave me her address, I knew exactly where it was.

Nevertheless, I was in. Like before, my sister and her (now) husband drove us. I still didn't have a driver's license or a car. When we drove up to her house, I thought I would die. It was all coming back. When I got to the door, and Mom opened it, I just wanted a hole to crawl into. I don't know whether my date knew anything about my family situation. She was nice all evening, and we had a good time. But I think she could sense I felt out of place.

I am still not much at small talk or glad-handing. I do seem to be able to appear far more at ease in such situations than I am. Friends and colleagues have often told me how they find it hard to believe I am shy and uncomfortable in these surroundings.

"I didn't want the night ever to end —and I couldn't wait for it to be over." *If you are reading this work, the above sentence made it through the various edits and re-writes. That's important to note. Reflecting on those days when life had such a small window of time to make comparisons, that statement still accurately reflects how I felt during those few hours. I remember feeling awkward, shy, embarrassed, and, simultaneously, like I was somebody! I can still see myself as if I had stepped out of my body and perused the room and the crowd. Looking at that reality from the outside, I did not want it to end. I wanted to belong. At that age, I was*

beginning to have a real sense of what "belonging" meant or required of one in life. I wanted to belong. Then, when I came back to reality, I just wanted to disappear. I wanted to be anywhere other than in the middle of a dark ballroom dance floor, surrounded by kids my age with whom it seemed I had nothing in common.

Now, all these years later, the issue is still unresolved. Sometimes, the moment is such that I never want it to end. Then comes the "I can't wait for this to be over" moment... or minutes, hours, days. That "small window of time within which to make comparisons" has grown. Twelve-fifteen years has become seventy-three years. How has the expansion of that window of time affected the comparison? I'm not sure. I think this grey-haired old man, with his 73-year frame of reference, is no more able to resolve this dilemma than that 13-year scaredy-cat on the ballroom floor.

As I go through this exercise and work through the memories and reflections, I repeatedly ask, "Why"? Why is all this such an issue? When I reflect on my growing-up years, they could have been much worse. Daddy left, and we had no money, but we were never on the streets. I was never unduly spanked or otherwise abused physically. Neither of my parents used alcohol or drugs (to my knowledge), not counting Mama's snuff-dipping). I never went hungry. Both parents lived many years past my growing-up years. So, why have I clung to this sense of fear and lack of self-worth? Without giving away the rest of the story, I did graduate from college. I married an incredible woman and fathered a fantastic son and daughter. I worked for 30 ½ years at the same college I graduated from. I have been blessed with better than reasonably good health. Why then? Why, then, during and after all these years, do I sometimes still wrestle with wanting the night/day never to end while simultaneously wishing it could all be over?

Chapter 5

NEVER GOOD ENOUGH

THE FALL OF 1964 arrived, and I was off to a new school and a new set of opportunities, adventures, failures, and disappointments. I was off as a sophomore to Goldsboro Senior High School. Later in my life, after "retiring" from my career working on a small college campus, I developed a mantra I used when working with college kids in a post-career mentoring program.:

FRIENDS - Choose them carefully, and cultivate;

CHOICES - Make them wisely, and learn:

CONSEQUENCES - Embrace them graciously, and move on!

I mention this now because, as I reflect on that transition to high school, I wish someone had recited those words to me then and pounded into my psyche their importance.

High school was little more than a continuation of the life I had come to know up to that point. I still lived in The Project. Papa still lived with us and was getting no better and no more likable. By now, my sister had graduated from high school, was married, moved out, and worked full-time. I still earned a little spending money in the summers working in tobacco on the farms of aunts and uncles. During these next three years, however, many changes would occur. I would assume greater responsibility at school, specifically as a manager and athletic trainer. I would get summer and weekend jobs that would put a little money in my pocket; not much, but more than I had ever known. I would begin to realize I could go to college. During a summer education program, I would have a life-changing experience that would introduce me to a new set of friends and a faith community with lifelong consequences. I would continue to experience life in two worlds. Sometimes those worlds confronted each other in painful ways.

The list of how these years were to be the same and then different goes on and on. Suffice it to say that I was excited to go to high school and had great expectations about it. While the days morphed into weeks, months, and years, I intuitively realized life's venues and accompanying noise were changing. But nothing of real consequence was changing. I still felt like a second-class citizen. I still felt like a failure. I still had no sense that I really mattered at all. I still remember my daddy's words, "I can't see through muddy water." I was working hard and making plans. I was doing well as a student. I had gained the trust and respect of teachers and coaches. But there were too many times in the quiet of a Saturday night at home with Mama and Papa or sitting in the back of a team bus on a late-night ride home, I still found myself asking the questions-Why? What difference does it all make? I would never be as good as Danny Davis, who lived on that stretch of Beech Street and would later go on to UNC as a Morehead Scholar, a scholarship for which I was nominated. I would never measure up to

Bud Andrews, whose sense of confidence and self-assurance I envied and whose family had a history of success and political engagement. I would never be good enough for Bailey Lowe's mother to approve of me, or for that matter, for Bailey to care for me the way I did her. What difference did it all make?

The transition was underway, and I was excited about it. Much of my high school years revolved around my role as Head Manager and athletic trainer for football, wrestling, and baseball. Time spent directly engaging in activities and some of the spin-offs resulting from them remain some of my life's best times to this day. I got into all that in junior high school when I realized I would not be big enough, strong enough, fast, or quick enough to be a good player in any of these sports. By working as a manager and then as the athletic trainer in high school, I found a way to be a "starter." The relationships those roles enabled me to have with players and coaches opened important doors then and continued to bless me in later years. My coaches placed a great deal of trust and confidence in me. I learned much about the importance of planning, organization, structure, reliability, and just plain old hard work and working smart. By junior year, I had keys to the entire field house, gym, and high school complex (everything but the principal's office). In keeping with the narrative herein, I now realize I must have missed out on untold opportunities that could materialize from these relationships. I missed out on them because of my fear of asking for help, for a favor, my fear of failure, and rejection. How might life have been different, better (or worse), had I been able to move outside that cocoon of fear and rejection? I'll never know. What difference does it really make now?

Reflecting on those years, I quickly realize my life today was molded by decisions made and the circles I lived and breathed in during that time- school and coaches, work at Wilber's Bar-B-Q, and those tobacco fields and barns. Choices made over the next fifty years can be traced back to conversations with a coach, a teacher, a schoolmate from that period, or a Quaker pastor who came into my life towards the end of that period. Nothing too unusual about this collection of influencers growing up. Many would argue that their lives were most affected by their friends and teachers encountered during their college years- if they attended college. I cannot say that those relationships did not strongly affect my life after college. In my journey, however, while the disruption may have been more pronounced during the college experience, the seeds for that disruption had their origin some years earlier in Goldsboro- never forgetting all this evolutionary tale repeatedly finds its way back to a little boy learning early in life that he was little more than "muddy water," and he should not "ask for a damn thing." Once again- FRIENDS-CHOICES-CONSEQUENCES! So, where to start?

It is hard to talk about any of this in any compartmentalized way. Coaches, teachers, and schoolmates all intermingle. And these all interact emotionally with The Project, Mama, and Papa. So, what follows will often reflect that emotional interaction. Let's give it a go and see where it leads.

My first introduction to Goldsboro High School (GHS) was through the football program. Due to my prior experience in junior high school, I arrived on campus at GHS, already plugged into the football scene and ready to work as a manager for the varsity as a sophomore. Usually, sophomores (10th graders) were relegated to the junior varsity. I got to start working with both. It was important to me. I felt special. The work was hard and sometimes very menial and dirty. But I was on the varsity team and contributing. The head coach was Gene Causby. He had been there for years. GHS had not had a good team in many years compared to some of the top 4-A programs across North Carolina. However, Coach Causby had raised the level of competitiveness, and the GHS Earthquakes were on the ascension. The fall of 1965, my sophomore year, was Coach Causby's final year as head coach. He would go on to have a significant career in secondary school and public-school administration at the state level. Coach Causby would be replaced the following year by one of his assistants, Gerald Whisenhunt, another Catawba College Indian. It was Coach Whisenhunt's first head coaching job.

My job as a manager meant getting to the new fieldhouse dressing room early and staying up late. My official boss was Coach Causby. My real boss was Tilly Hanson, or Dr. "T," as he was called. Dr. T had graduated the previous spring after being a manager and athletic trainer for three years. Somehow, Coach Causby found money to hire Dr. T for the football season. Dr. T was in charge. He was a stern taskmaster. He knew what needed to be done and expected it to be done well and on time. The last thing he wanted was Coach Causby calling him because something was not where it was supposed to be when it was supposed to be there. I proved to be teachable and willing to learn. I loved it. I loved it. I loved it. Apparently, I curried the favor of Dr. T and Coach Causby early on. Not too far into the season, Dr. T began to bring me under his wing and include me in some of his duties as the athletic trainer. I was being groomed to take on that role the next year. As it turned out, I was not the only one being groomed for the next year. Little did we know then, but Coach Whisenhunt (Coach Whis) would replace Coach Causby the next year as he moved on to be principal at the junior high school.

That fall of 1964 was the most beautiful four months of my young life up to that point. I was out of the house more. I was being given a role of responsibility and accomplishing it well. Further, I was exposed to a world with little prior experience. While my junior high school years allowed me to ride the roads of eastern North Carolina, high school football added a new dimension. We played a more extensive schedule on Friday nights. We had practice every school day. The coaches also met on Saturday mornings to review film from the night before. To assist in that duty, Dr. T and the managers were there to get the previous night's uniforms to the cleaners, clean the dressing room, and prepare for Monday's practice. One of our most important jobs on Saturday mornings was to visit Mickey's Pastry Shop next door to the cleaners. Mickey McClenny, a Quaker and lifelong member of Goldsboro Friends Meeting, owned the best local pastry shop in eastern North Carolina and was a staunch supporter of the Earthquakes. He was also an NCAA football official. So, every Saturday morning during football season, we would stop in the shop after depositing our load at the cleaners and pick up a box of day-old doughnuts of various shapes and sizes. We were on our honor to get them to the coach's office in time for their meeting. That we did, for the most part. Usually, some of the inventory would get lost along the way. The coaches never called us out on it. They knew. It was just one of the benefits of the job. Some of that routine would change the following year after Dr. T left to join the Coast Guard and I was placed in charge. Much would stay the same. Dr. T had been a good teacher. There was no need to change much.

The routine during football season became clear. I was fortunate to have arrived on the scene when a brand-new field house facility opened for use. I didn't have any basis for comparing our new digs with other high schools in our world. All I knew was that we had a nice place to call home. Once we started making road trips, I discovered that we indeed had a very nice and functional place to call home. The building opened that year. It was nearly as long as the field was wide. It sat just a few feet outside the fence behind the west endzone. At one end was a small coach's office with a private shower facility. Next to that was the training room with a training table, a whirlpool, and adequate storage space for medical supplies. I would have an exciting time during the season and subsequent seasons decorating the wall with pictures of favorite NFL players from Sports Illustrated magazine. Players from our team would bring pictures of their favorites to put on the walls. The training room became a focal point of activity before and after practices. The rest of this central part of the facility was the dressing room with open lockers and bathroom and shower space sufficient for our numbers.

Dr. T had keys to the building so he could get us managers into the space whenever we needed to be there before the arrival of the players and on weekends if necessary. I would inherit those keys and more the following year after Dr. T's departure. Next to the dressing room was a bigger room. It was big enough to accommodate a full-size competition-grade wrestling mat that could be rolled up and transported to the basketball gym for official matches. Otherwise, during wrestling season, which came along right after football, it stayed rolled open on the floor in that room. However, during football, it stayed rolled up along one side of the floor. At the far end of the wrestling room was a caged storage room with a garage-type door that opened to the outside. That is where all the football equipment was stored. There we kept the extra individual gear: practice and game uniforms, shoulder and hip pads, helmets, replacement cleats, etc. We also kept any surplus medical supplies whenever we ran out of room in the training room. Finally, it was where we stored the huge blocking dummies and pads used in practice every day. That was the one part of the job I dreaded. I weighed only 149 pounds during high school, maybe even less when I first arrived. Those blocking dummies were as big as I was and weighed more. As managers, our job was to move these things from the storage cage to the practice field daily and back into the cage after practice. Using a wheelbarrow and trying to balance it was hard work. It was hard enough on a good day, almost impossible when it rained. Rain did not stop practice, usually. The rest of the building provided space for a band practice room, a dressing room, coach's offices, and a dressing room for the baseball team. For the next two years, this was MY domain- my home away from home. The Project might as well have been a million miles away.

I cannot let this pass. Dr. T was fastidious in every way. He was always a neat dresser. He oversaw the dress code for us managers. On game nights, we wore long sleeve white coveralls with sufficient pockets and loops to accommodate all the replacement equipment pieces and, in the case of the trainer, medical paraphernalia. After every practice, the dressing room had to be swept and cleared of all dirty laundry. There was a washer and dryer across the parking lot in the janitor's HQ, where we would take towels and practice uniforms to launder. That laundry room became my "go-to" place when I needed to get away. The janitor, Alonzo Cherry, had been the high school janitor for many years, and everybody loved him. Few students got to know him as I did, though. Many days, either during or after practice, I would take a load of things across the parking lot to the laundry room, and there would be Mr. Cherry. When he had the time, he would stay and linger. We had many great talks in the solitude of that damp, hot, noisy laundry room. Whenever I needed anything, Mr. Cherry could be counted on to help me find it. Many day-old donuts found their way to Alonzo's crib. Over the years, I have wished I could have known him better. I think we could have become good friends.

Back to Dr. T. Dr. T was particular about his car. Right around the start of the season, he bought a brand-new VW Beetle. It was a beautiful green color. It was the first car Dr. T had ever owned. He was so proud of it. I would have been too. Don't ask me how this came about. I honestly don't remember. I have been told over the years that I was the plot's mastermind. Maybe! I really don't remember. It went something like this. Dr. T occasionally parked his prized possession right outside the garage doors to the storage cage, between the building and the fence to the field. There was just enough room for it to fit in there. He liked to protect it from errant traffic on the parking lot side of the building. He didn't do this all the time, just occasionally. He was called away from the facility for something on one such occasion. It was not unusual for a coach to send him on an "official" errand. On this occasion, by the time he returned, practice was over, the coaches were gone, and almost all the players had left. When Dr. T went outside to get into his car- it was not there. It was gone. He walked all around the building and through the parking lot. He made sure he had the keys in his pocket. He was beside himself. The only people still there were me, the other managers, and three or four players hanging around. Dr. T went ballistic. He could have a temper sometime. When he went off, he could cuss like I had never heard before. This quickly became one such time. After a while, when he was convinced the car was nowhere to be found, he headed off to the coach's office to call the police. Remember, this was 1964; there were no cell phones yet. Before he could dial the number for the police, I managed to stop him. I could not let him call the cops. I got him to put the phone down and come with me. We walked through the wrestling room to the equipment storage cage.

Suddenly, I feared for my life. Behind the locked cage door, surrounded by a zoo of football gear, sat Dr. T's beautiful green, shiny Beetle, smiling up at him like a lost child. Dr. T's first reaction was joy and relief. That only lasted a moment. It was followed by an explosion. I thought he would kill me as if I was responsible. Had it not been for the other managers and players standing around, he might have. While Dr. T was away and after the coaches had left, someone raised the garage door to the cage, and several teenage boys banded together to lift that beautiful child and place it in the cage, never unlocking the inside cage door. Once discovered, the car had to be removed just like it had been placed in the cage. There was not enough room to turn it to drive it out. Once the car was out and Dr. T confirmed there were no scratches or marks on it, he calmed down just a little; enough so we could finish our few remaining tasks in the dressing room and go home. Dr. T made it abundantly clear that if anyone ever touched his baby again, it might be the last thing they ever touched. I learned that lesson well. I never touched his baby again. Those years, and the subsequent initial college years, might have been less harrowing (and less interesting) had I taken that advice to heart in other arenas.

The remainder of that year, 1964-65, was spent learning the ropes and making new friends. I did well academically and began believing there was a place for me. After football season, I spent much of my time outside class in the fieldhouse. I worked as the manager for the wrestling team. It was in that capacity that I got to know Coach Whis better. He was an assistant coach for football. He would become the head coach the next year. He also coached the wrestling team and track and field. I was to become his number-one student assistant year-round. By the time school started the next fall, he was Head Coach and I was the Head Manager and trainer. That show of trust made a huge impact on me. Over the years, I have regretted that I didn't fully grasp the importance of that trust and appreciate it as sincerely as I should have. I was an inexperienced kid, perhaps ill-prepared for the responsibility I was given. I did a good job in my assigned duties. There's no argument about that. I failed to understand the inherent boundaries associated with that responsibility.

I wanted to be liked. I tried to fit in. I never did anything life-threatening or much outside the bounds of most high school brats. I wandered outside the lines. Chalk it up to a typical teenager pushing the envelope. I don't know. All I know is that during this year, I was changing. I was still excelling in the classroom and assuming a role of responsibility, albeit behind the scenes in many ways. Somehow, I think I still wanted to be "somebody." That struggle to be "somebody" would dog me the rest of my life. Even when successful in the small niche I claimed for myself, I always felt like I was not "good enough" when I compared myself to the doctors, the lawyers, the business owners, and the Morehead Scholars. I was constantly trying to measure up.

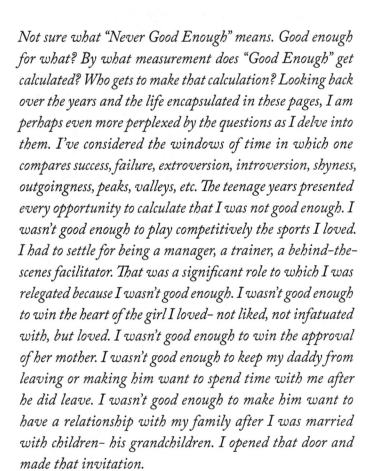

Not sure what "Never Good Enough" means. Good enough for what? By what measurement does "Good Enough" get calculated? Who gets to make that calculation? Looking back over the years and the life encapsulated in these pages, I am perhaps even more perplexed by the questions as I delve into them. I've considered the windows of time in which one compares success, failure, extroversion, introversion, shyness, outgoingness, peaks, valleys, etc. The teenage years presented every opportunity to calculate that I was not good enough. I wasn't good enough to play competitively the sports I loved. I had to settle for being a manager, a trainer, a behind-the-scenes facilitator. That was a significant role to which I was relegated because I wasn't good enough. I wasn't good enough to win the heart of the girl I loved– not liked, not infatuated with, but loved. I wasn't good enough to win the approval of her mother. I wasn't good enough to keep my daddy from leaving or making him want to spend time with me after he did leave. I wasn't good enough to make him want to have a relationship with my family after I was married with children– his grandchildren. I opened that door and made that invitation.

Is the meaning of "good enough" really this simple? Or much more complicated? Can one's failure to be good enough be a misinterpretation of another person's assessment of one's status? Perhaps the ground rules have been misjudged, misapplied. Who gets to make that assessment? How did I allow my behavior to be guided by how I thought someone else saw me? I don't know. Does it matter who is at fault?

Perhaps. All I know is that somewhere in those early years leading up to the pre-teens and high school years, I learned that, on many fronts, I was not good enough. That learned, I was rarely ever able to act outside of that internalized belief. Belief or fact, the effect was the same. As a result, I will never know the doors I failed to open and opportunities I failed to realize simply because I entered the fray, having already decided I was "never good enough" and never strong enough to ask for help!

Chapter 6

OUTSIDE LOOKING IN

I DON'T KNOW how to describe the final two years of high school. High school was then and still is (maybe even more so) a time of diverging growth patterns and developing priorities. I can say without hesitation that those two years were, at one moment, the most exciting and inspiring times of my life: then, at another moment, the most depressing and anger-inducing times of my life, assuming a role of significant responsibility inside the athletic arena, albeit from behind the scenes in a purely supportive role. I was not a star athlete. Hell- I wasn't an athlete at all.

Nevertheless, my sense of belonging and leadership derived from my head manager and athletic trainer role. My teachers recognized me as a top student and student leader. I don't know how much they knew about my home life. The coaches knew something about it, although I wonder how they knew. The final two years of high school began, and I couldn't wait for life to unfold. I was excited to get up in the morning and head off to school, anticipating what the day held in store. I had no idea when and how profoundly a sense of "living on the outside looking in" would engulf me.

These years were full of life and adventures. Papa was still with us. I still had my duties at home, helping Mama with him. I hate to admit it. I had grown to resent his presence and the demands it placed on Mama and me to some extent. Other than Glenn Aycock, I never had any friends over to visit. Even then, Glenn was there for one reason only. He never ventured beyond the small living room and kitchen, where we would sit to help with his homework. I was embarrassed about where and how we lived. I don't know what role Papa played in triggering that embarrassment. It doesn't matter. I felt it, and it was real. Over the years, I have regretted how I felt about Papa. It wasn't his fault how I felt.

As I have looked back and tried to revisit those years, I have realized he had little to do with it. I was a poor kid whose daddy wanted another woman more than he wanted his son. I could be among the smartest kids in the school and well-liked by others from all striations in the social spectrum. When I found myself alone or at home in that apartment in The Project, I often felt like I was only looking in from the outside as life moved along. Now, as I have grown older and gotten to know more of the stories of some of my classmates, and my fellow Earthquakes, I have gained a better appreciation of the fact that I was not the only kid living with challenging life situations. On the other hand, I have continued to experience the same "never good enough" and "outside looking in" feelings as I have seen others achieve positions of accomplishment and financial success I find myself envying- coveting. I hate the feeling that I must be the biggest underachiever ever- indeed, the biggest underachiever to come through those years in that place.

Well, let's look at some of the specifics of those years. Most of what I remember and believe impacted my life most significantly revolved around time spent at school or school-sponsored events, particularly athletic events. During the summers, my time was primarily spent working at Wilber's Bar-B-Q or in tobacco on relatives' farms. Where to begin? Let's talk about tobacco first. I mentioned previously that while my immediate family lived in Goldsboro, all my aunts and uncles farmed in the country. From the time I was a small child (five years old or so), I had been around the barning of tobacco. Mama would take me with her when she worked on one of these farms during the summer tobacco harvesting season. As I grew older, I could also work, first handing the tobacco leaves from a trailer to someone, usually, my mama, who would attach the leaves to a long stick using string- tobacco twine. The tobacco would be placed in a large barn where it would cure using small oil burners. When I got big enough, during junior high school, I learned how to drive a tractor, and I could drive the trailers in the fields where the tobacco leaves were being "cropped" and take them to the shelters where they would be "strung" onto the tobacco sticks. Later, when I reached high school age and size, I could work either inside the barn, hanging the sticks after they were strung, or working in the fields, cropping tobacco- breaking the leaves from their stalks and placing them in the trailer. Each of these steps up the job ladder carried with it a slightly higher hourly wage. By the time I was in high school, I was working three to four days a week during the harvesting season, either cropping or hanging. [I used to joke with friends that I was so excited when high school graduation was approaching. I was going to college and would never have to go into another tobacco patch or hang another stick of tobacco. Little did I know that I would meet the cutest student nurse I had ever seen four years later, and she would happen to be the farmer's daughter.]

Working in tobacco was hard, dirty work. I hated every minute of it. The pay wasn't much. It was something, though, and I didn't have many choices then. I might have had more options if I had only asked. Back to the fear of asking for help. It did put a little spending money in my pocket. Mama never asked me to give her any of my earnings. Mama never made me feel like I had to help support the household. She had no money to give me, but I could keep what I earned. All together I worked on the farms of two uncles, one cousin, and the cousin of our next-door neighbor. One of the uncles was married to mama's sister. Aunt Laulas was the oldest of my aunts. She and Uncle Walter were two of the few aunts and uncles who came to visit us and see Papa. I know they helped a little financially as well.

I worked in their tobacco harvesting for two summers, between my junior and senior year and after graduating. When we didn't have tobacco to harvest, Uncle Walter would get me to do other odd jobs around the farm. I remember vividly the joys of mending the fencing around the pig pens and walking acres of soybeans to pull weeds. I will never forget Aunt Laulas coming to get me from the field to tell me Papa had passed away. It was the summer I had just graduated from high school, July 13, 1967. Years later, Mama would note she had worried about how she would go about taking care of Papa when I went off to college. She was convinced God took him that summer, knowing she couldn't care for him without my help.

One of my good memories about working with Uncle Walter and Aunt Laulas was lunch. Aunt Laulas was an excellent cook. Most farm wives were/are. While we were out "putting in tobacco," she prepared a full lunch. We would have fried chicken or meatloaf, a country-fried steak, at least two vegetables, usually stewed potatoes or rice, maybe green beans, and homemade fresh-from-scratch biscuits. She would always have some dessert, usually a fruit pie. Virtually everything came from the farm- the meat, the vegetables, and much of the fruit. They bought the rice and the flour. It was hard going back to work after that kind of meal. Uncle Walter and Aunt Laulas were truly kind to me and mama. They were interesting, funny, and Aunt Laulas was a hard worker- not so much Uncle Walter. He was a bit unorganized and, some would say, lazy. Aunt Laulas, on the other hand, was a worker, organized, focused, and tirelessly committed to whatever the task was. They made a good living for themselves. Judging from outward appearances, they may have been the most well-heeled of all my relatives. I have no way of knowing.

I have one memory of my time working on those tobacco farms, and Uncle Walter and Aunt Laulas specifically. We must remember here I am talking about life in the South in the 1960s. By the summer of 1965, school desegregation had been adopted as law. It was, however, far from being the actual law of the land. I had never been around Black folks; had never lived near any; had never been to school with any (although I do remember our first Black students coming to GHS during my junior year); had certainly never sat at a dining table with any. I had grown up hearing the word 'nigger,' and 'darkie.' I must confess, though, that I have no memory of using those words. Given their regular appearance when around extended family, I don't know why. Perhaps my affinity for George Washington Carver. the tobacco fields and barns. Where I worked in tobacco, most workers were family members or Black folks. The summer of 1967 at Uncle Walter and Aunt Laulas' was the same, with one difference. On the days when we had no tobacco work, Uncle

Walter would come to get me. He would also pick up one older teenage Black kid. I do not remember his name, just that he was a little older than me and certainly bigger and stronger. He was not very talkative but polite enough. We worked together on whatever project Uncle Walter assigned to us. We got along fine. When lunchtime came, we went to the house to wash up and eat. Aunt Laulas fixed the Black boy a plate, and he ate in the yard, sitting near the back door. Uncle Walter, Aunt Laulas, and I enjoyed lunch at their dining room table.

I have never gotten over the shame of not addressing that situation at the time. I could have appealed to my relatives to allow the boy to join us, which I am sure they would not have done. I could be wrong. Who knows how they might have reacted? They might have kicked me out, also. I'll never know. Or, I could have excused myself and joined him outside. Either one would have been better than saying or doing nothing. Uncle Walter and Aunt Laulas were good people. They behaved as they had been trained all their lives to behave. Due to my experience in Barbourville the previous summer, I knew in my heart that the eating separation was not right. I also knew it would not be well received by my relatives if I spoke up about it. So, I never broached the subject, and the boy and I never talked about it. I've often wondered whatever happened to him. I've wondered if, at the time, he ever considered making an issue of it or asking me about it. Or, had he been so indoctrinated all his life that he never considered the slight we all were imposing on him?

Early in my junior year, I was fortunate to get a part-time job at Wilber's Bar-B-Q. My friend, Glenn Aycock, attended church with Mr. Wilber Shirley, owner of the BBQ restaurant, and had worked there since he was old enough to have a work permit. Glenn knew I wanted a job; He asked Wilber if he could use another kid, and Wilber said sure. So, soon after school started, I found myself busing tables at Wilber's on Saturdays and Sundays. I also worked occasional parties Wilber was catering. It was fun work for the most part, and the pay was OK. I was also assured a free BBQ lunch on days I worked.

Wilber's was known everywhere as one of the preeminent BBQ establishments in North Carolina. Located on Hwy 70 just east of Goldsboro near Seymour Johnson AFB, it was a favorite stopping place for weekend beach traffic and vacationers heading to or from Morehead City and Atlantic Beach. We were always busy. I'll always remember the day I got promoted from busboy to waiter. It was a busy Sunday lunchtime, and I was hustling to keep tables cleared and clean. I was walking by a table of four older ladies who had been seated. No one had taken their orders, and Wilber was anxious to have them served. It was near the front, just down from the front door and cashier's station. Wilber was standing nearby doing his usual meet-and-greet thing. He noticed the ladies had been seated for a few minutes, and no one had arrived to serve them. As I walked by on my way to unload my dishes from the table I had just cleared, Wilber stopped me and told me to get rid of my load and come back and "wait on that table." I was frozen in my tracks. I had never waited on a table. My immediate response to Wilber was, "I don't have an order pad or pen," thinking that would get me off the hook. Wilber came back. "Find a pad and grab a muddy stick if you have to, but go get their order." When my heart started beating again, I did as ordered. I ran to the kitchen to offload my dishes. I found an order pad and grabbed a pen from the cashier's station. Hence, my promotion and increase in pay were launched. I remember being so nervous that I could hardly breathe. I did introduce myself to the ladies and took their orders. I got them served in a reasonable time. I must have done OK because I remember my first tip- it was a good one. I worked at Wilber's until I left for college. I will be forever grateful for the job Wilber gave me and to Glenn for making that introduction.

On a side note, working at Wilber's is where I gained driving experience. I turned sixteen in October of my junior year. There was no car in our home. My sister was married by then. I did take driver's training (Coach Whis was my driving instructor). I passed. My sister let me use her car to take my driving test to get my license. It was a big Pontiac Bonneville. I was scared to drive it, but I did, and I got my license. Now, I had a license and nothing to drive. At closing time at the restaurant, the chief cook, a delightfully older Black lady, had to be driven home. Wilber had an old, early fifties, red Ford pick-up truck used for hauling pig stock and waste products. Someone had to take the truck and "drive Ms. Daisey" home each night. I always volunteered for this duty. Often, I would get the nod. I was in heaven. This old truck was a three-speed straight drive with gears on the column (3 on the tree) and a starter pedal on the floor. That is where I learned how to drive.

Wilber Shirley gave me a real job that was not in a tobacco patch. He trusted me to drive one of his most valued employees home in a vehicle he owned. I have continued to see Wilber over the years. Rarely have I returned to Goldsboro for family or GHS reunion visits that I have not enjoyed some good ole Wilber's BBQ. Until the last few years, Wilber continued to be on the scene, meeting and greeting.

Let me digress a little- back again to the start of my junior year. Before school started, football was well underway. The previous head coach, Gene Causby, and the new head coach, Gerald Whisenhunt, were graduates of Catawba College in Salisbury, NC. Both had stellar athletic records there and had made lifelong friends and connections in the Salisbury community. One of those connections led them to the Kiwanis Health Camp. This was a "retreat"-type facility just outside Salisbury. A central building housed a kitchen and a large, open dining and meeting area. There were two long bunk rooms, each equipped to sleep about thirty or so guys. There were also three or four smaller, more private bedrooms. Outside the building was the usual wooded area, surrounded by an ample open space- The Hill. The Hill was a space about the size of a football field. Rather than being flat, it had a pronounced slope in all four directions. It really was- The Hill. The location was far enough from town and surrounded by woods with a long dirt driveway. It was secluded.

Before school started, the football team- coaches, players, managers, and trainer, tackling sleds and dummies- everybody and everything- boarded buses and a truck to spend two weeks at Camp. I don't know how the coaches managed to secure funding and insurance for this off-campus two-week preseason camp. Eventually, cost and other administrative roadblocks brought it to an end. For now, however, we were going to football camp. For two weeks, there was practice in full pads at six o'clock in the morning. Players requiring taping or some other medical care had to be in the trainer's station in advance. Needing this kind of pre-practice attention was no excuse for being late to practice. Breakfast followed. Skull sessions (film and play reviews) were next. At noon there was practice in shorts, shirts, and helmets. The goal was to work on learning plays and practicing kickoffs and punts.

After this 'light' practice, there was lunch and a mail call. After the mail call, there was afternoon R&R. At five o'clock, we were back on The Hill in full gear. Again, medical attention before practice was no excuse for being late. These two weeks were in mid-August. It was hot and humid. Supper followed this late afternoon session. After supper, everyone gathered for another skull session. After these sessions, I would see anyone needing further medical attention- icing, rubdowns, heat treatments, etc. By the time we finished it was lights out. Then, a few hours later, coaches would appear, blowing their whistles, and we would do it all again. This was the daily schedule, Monday through Saturday, for two weeks. There were NO visitors or phone calls during the week. The Sunday between the two weeks was Visitors Day. By the end of the first week, everybody looked forward to the arrival of families, girlfriends, and cheerleaders on Sunday. The day passed too quickly. I had no family come, and I didn't have a girlfriend to share the day with. I used the day to catch up on organizing equipment, laundry, and prepping for the second week. There was always a handful of players requiring attention, even on Sunday. After everyone left, we all had supper, followed by another skull session. Monday morning arrived bright and early, and it all began again.

Those days were hard, dirty, and sweaty. The Hill was not a pristine grassy slope. There was grass- some grass. It was sparse, with plenty of bare spots. Players were bruised and banged up by week's end. Tempers would flare. Hey, it was football camp. The theme song for the Camp was The Animals' "House of the Rising Sun," which was released in 1964. Somehow, it just seemed to set the tone.

Why have I taken this much time and space to describe what was, after all, just a couple of two-week experiences with coaches and players? Perhaps nothing in my high school experience better personifies my "outside looking in" feelings. For two weeks, we were a team together, working to accomplish something that no team in the history of GHS had ever accomplished. We had the talent and the coaching to be the best football team over the next two years that GHS had ever seen. During the practice sessions, that was all the focus. After the sessions, when players and coaches were coming down from the immediately preceding events, I was busy cleaning up, searching for lost footballs in the woods next to the practice field, or getting ready for the next practice session. I sometimes had to take a manager with me to a nearby shopping mall to find a laundromat to catch up on laundry needs. It was during these moments that it would sometimes hit me. I was never going to be a part of the team and share in its successes, unlike dressed-out players. I would always be the guy who arrived early to prep and stayed late to clean up and get equipment back to its place. I would always be the guy who carried water to the guys who were running, sweating, and getting banged up. What I did was important. But anybody could do it. I could have been replaced, and no one would have ever missed me. You couldn't so easily replace those guys with numbers on their backs. I would never know what it felt like to be "that guy." I would always be outside looking into "that guy's" life and wishing. Over the years, this team has had a remarkable record of staying together. We have had reunions, and we stay in touch with the help of social media. Some of us have attended funerals and memorial services. After fifty years, a group of nearly twenty of us with two coaches visited what was the Kiwanis Health Camp and stood atop The Hill. The members of that team have always treated me like a full member of the team. I am deeply appreciative of that. But I know, and I knew then, the success of that team never depended much on what I did. Someone else could have easily taken over my role. Even third-string players who rode the bench were more critical to the actual success of the team. They worked hard during these two weeks and later every day after school in practice. Their working and pushing the starters made the starters better. I am not having a pity party here. I'm not shortchanging the value of what I did. I'm acknowledging what I believe to be a fact; I saw my role as a second-class citizen when I desperately wanted to be first-class. Right or wrong, justified or not, that is how I found myself looking at things back then, in those moments when my mind was not otherwise focused. That is how I have looked at life for most of these seventy years.

Returning from Camp, we launched full speed ahead into the school year. Classes were good. Football progressed well. For the first time in years, perhaps ever, the Goldsboro Earthquakes were showing in statewide newspaper rankings in the Top-10. Since I was now the head manager and trainer, I launched a new practice. With permission from Coach Whis, I and the other managers would spend Friday nights in the fieldhouse after football games. We used the time to clean the locker room and showers. I tidied up the training room. The following day, we made the laundry run and picked up the donuts from Mickey's.

Those were our official duties on those nights. That is not all that took place. I had a great staff. Rarely did we sleep much on those nights. Occasionally we would be joined by a player or two from the team. On more than one occasion, we would walk over to the main school facility and visit the Home Ec room and cafeteria kitchen. We could always find something good to eat in one place or the other. In the Home Ec room, we found cake made by classmates. We never knew who. We did appreciate their efforts. I've often wondered if the teacher or students ever wondered what was happening with cake leftovers in their freezer. I hope no one ever pointed their finger at my friend, Alonzo, the janitor. [I never thought about that possibility until now]. We often found leftover chocolate peanut butter delights in the cafe kitchen. The head dietician was the same lady who went to Camp with the football team, Ms. Edgerton. I had not been introduced to the local Quaker Meeting at that time. It turns out she was also a member of that church. Anyway, we ate well on those nights.

I must confess there was never any alcohol involved in those nights. I didn't drink, and I knew that any hint of such would be the end of that freedom if it got back to Coach Whis. (Funny how it never occurred to me to equate the potential loss of that freedom (not to mention being kicked from the team and maybe suspended from school) with both drinking and raiding the school. On one occasion, another of my good friends, perhaps my best friend in high school, Bud Andrews, stayed with us for a good portion of the night. Sometime during the night, we drove over to the house of a girl he dated occasionally, whom we both "loved dearly." When she awoke the following day, she walked out to a beautifully and generously "forked" yard. Bud and I both denied having anything to do with it. She knew!

All home football games, and weekend home basketball games, were followed by a sock hop in the school gym or a dance at the St. Stephens Parish House. I looked forward to these times. Unfortunately, I was still painfully shy and rarely had a date for either of these events. But hope sprang eternally. I could always get a ride when the dance was at the Parish House.

I didn't dance much- way too shy to ask. I was there, and most guys and girls there were without dates. It wasn't until later in my senior year that I had anything resembling a regular date. On balance, those were good times.

After football season, I continued spending as much time in the fieldhouse as possible. I was the manager and trainer for the wrestling team. Like the football program, the GHS wrestling program was on the ascent. We won the regional championship that year and made a run at state. When spring arrived, I stayed on as manager and trainer for the track and field team. Track and field had received little attention at GHS. There was little funding for it and virtually no physical facilities, other than a run-down track around an open field at the junior high school.

Nevertheless, I showed up to do my job. My heart was never in it. I owed it to Coach Whis though. By the time we were midway through the spring sports season, I was much more interested in the baseball season. I would move from track to working for the baseball team in my senior year.

While athletic seasons were unfolding, I was doing well in school. I was selected to be a Junior Marshall. That was a serious academic honor, awarded to only the top 25 students in the junior class. Our job was to serve as receptionists and ushers at events held in the school auditorium and open to the public concerts, plays, and special speakers. I was honored to be in that group. I was proud. I somehow knew I belonged there academically. I had to buy a formal suit to wear for these events. It was a formal suit with a white tuxedo. I have no idea how Mama and I found the money to pay for such a thing. It was the most expensive wearing apparel ever to find its way to 801-A Taylor Street. Whenever we worked an event, I looked at the other marshals, particularly the girls, and thought how incredibly handsome and beautiful we were. I wanted desperately to summon the courage to ask some of them out on a date. I never did. I can't describe how it felt.

When the events were over and the crowds were gone, our job was done. We would be excused to go home. And home I went, walking back to The Project, usually late at night. Neither Bud nor Glenn were marshals. I wouldn't ask anyone else for a lift. I was never afraid to walk home. But it always happened by the time I had walked a block or two from the school. That warm, happy feeling I had experienced just a couple of hours earlier would begin to fade. Before I knew it, I was going to that place I dreaded. Once again, I was on the outside looking in. I could do well in school and wear an expensive tux, but I would never belong. I would always walk back to The Project by myself.

Sometime during the early spring semester of my junior year, I received a note from an assistant football coach that would redirect my life's direction forever. Coach Sam Shugart would open a door that I willingly went through. Coach Shugart called me into his office one day. In addition to being an assistant football coach, Coach Shugart was an assistant principal. You can imagine. I was scared when I got the message he wanted to see me. I thought someone had found out about our Friday visits to the Home Ec room and the cafe kitchen. Well, that wasn't it—quite the contrary. Coach Shugart was one to be feared, and, at the same time, he had a keen sense of humor. Coach was well known for his mantra to linemen during practices: you gotta be "Agile, Mobile, and Hostile." At this moment, his less-threatening side was about to be displayed. He wanted to know if I might be interested in going to Kentucky the upcoming summer. Before knowing anything about what he was offering,

I said, "Yes." He explained that a local businessman, Wilbur Roberts, was financially sponsoring one student to attend a six-week on-campus program in Barbourville, KY. The Encampment for Citizenship was housed at Union College in Barbourville in Knox County, the heart of Appalachian coal country. The Encampment was a summer encampment experience that would bring together 120 high school kids from across America- Black, White, Hispanic, Native American, rich, poor, urban, and rural. Scholarship funds were available so they could bring together kids from all economic strata. A well-known local businessman was providing 100% of the cost, including the bus ticket and $5 a week spending money. Five dollars a week doesn't sound like much now. In 1966 it was OK. The program was run out of its headquarters in New York City. Eleanor Roosevelt was one of the founders. The mission of the Encampment was a sociological experiment.

Bring together these 120 high school kids from across the sociological spectrum. Have them live together in college dorms. Share meals. Take classes and field trips together. Spend time together on campus, in the lounges, and on the trails. Live together for a week in the "hollers" with families who lived there. I had no idea what I was getting into. I was the only student from North Carolina. I shared a dorm room for six weeks with a Jewish kid from New York City and a 6'6" tall Black kid from Alabama. I didn't sleep for a week. My life and how I saw the world was about to change. The school year ended, and I was full of anticipation. I had a good weekend gig at Wilber's and all the work I wanted in the tobacco fields. Football camp would be here before you knew it. And, in between, I was going out of state for the first time. Little did I know what lay ahead.

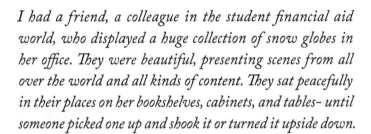

I had a friend, a colleague in the student financial aid world, who displayed a huge collection of snow globes in her office. They were beautiful, presenting scenes from all over the world and all kinds of content. They sat peacefully in their places on her bookshelves, cabinets, and tables- until someone picked one up and shook it or turned it upside down.

I have another friend, also from the student financial aid world. She is one of the quietest, calmest, most mild-mannered people I've ever met. That is until she climbs onto a roller coaster. Then she goes berserk like a bat out of hell. I don't do roller coasters. I just don't ride them. I'll jump out of a perfectly good airplane but do not put me on a coaster. I have had occasion to see her at work on one. She morphs into something, someone I would never recognize in real life.

When I think about it, I have lived much of my life looking into a snow globe. I have seen some beautiful things and witnessed some incredible moments. But, for the most part, I have been an innocent observer, looking through the globe, too afraid to participate in its adventures. Other times, when I dared reach out to touch the globe, often the experience amounted to little more than watching through the snow. As a result, I've rarely climbed into the scene and enjoyed the snowfall.

I suppose I must admit I have occasionally climbed onto that roller coaster. It's a funny thing. But, as I reflect and try to recapture those moments, I am discovering that when I have climbed aboard, somehow overcoming the fear or managing to "find a way" to inject myself into the scene, the result has almost always been good. There may be temporary discomforts and wishing otherwise sometimes. Usually, though, the fears have been unfounded, and the results worth the effort required to find a way into the globe or jump onto the coaster.

Even now, coming down the backstretch of life and working through this reflective exercise, confessing I can understand that the rare diving into the globe and climbing aboard the coaster moments may have been worth the efforts, I still cannot understand why I have lived life this way. I am sure, as the days, the weeks, the years of life unfolded, and I faced the daily events of life, it never occurred to me that I was living outside the globe, looking in. I never considered living life as a spectator, aching to climb aboard the coaster. Looking back, I recall a multitude of times, places, and events where my heart ached because I was on the outside looking in, where I wanted so badly to take that exhilarating ride, but either wouldn't because I was afraid to take the step, or didn't because I couldn't "find a way" in or on.

Now, approaching my mid-70s, the opportunities to jump into the globe or climb aboard the coaster seem to dwindle. I have never had a lot of friends- real friends. I've always had a lot of acquaintances; due to the nature of the kinds of work or activities I have pursued. Had I been more engaging, I might have had a more extensive network of real friends at this stage of my life. I didn't, so I don't. It's too late to do much about that. The irony of all this perplexes me: I wish I had lived inside the globe and jumped onto the coaster more readily. I would have more social engagement today.

On the other hand, I am perfectly happy in my solitude – or am I? I am OK being alone, if I am alone within the context of a place I know and love and I know Becky is near, or soon will be. Sometimes I wish I had made better work and financial decisions throughout life; so that now Becky and I could enjoy more of the things we like to do. I suppose that is the wish of most older men. In my case, I do believe it could have been different had I lived up to the level of ability and performance of which I was capable. Back to the same old issue: I never could ask for anything, including help, when I needed help, and I never felt worthy of asking anyone to go out of their way to provide that help. So, here we are. The days, the weeks, the years are still passing by, seemingly at a faster pace than ever before. Although now recognizing those issues and putting names to them, nothing much has changed. The peaks and the valleys– they still occur. Mostly, the days and weeks just come, and they go.

Chapter 7

INTRODUCTION TO QUAKERISM

THE SUMMER OF 1966 came, and I was all about getting ready for my bus trip to Union College in Barbourville, KY. The six-week program was to run from mid-June to the end of July. My sister Joyce, and Mama, took me to the bus station late in the afternoon to catch a Greyhound bus that would get me there mid-afternoon the next day. It was an uncomfortable all-night ride, one I had waited for with great expectations. But I would not be disappointed. I arrived in Barbourville and was met at the bus station by a staff person from the Encampment. By day's end, I was in my dorm room. I met my two roommates whom I mentioned previously. In the interest of time, I will not cover these six weeks in detail. There is just too much there. Instead, I will relate a few specific events during this time as they directly impacted my future developments and choices.

I described the basic makeup of this gathering of 120 high school kids from around the country. It is important to note where the country was in the summer of 1966. The war in Vietnam was raging, and the anti-war, anti-draft movement was gathering steam. The Civil Rights movement was well underway. Riots were taking place across the country. The Watts section of Los Angeles had been ablaze the previous year. One of the kids in the program was an outspoken Black kid from Watts. He had been on the streets in the middle of it all. The "war on poverty" enacted by Congress under President Lyndon Johnson's leadership was taking shape and gathering soldiers. The mission of the Encampment was to pull together this microcosm of American youth and see how we would interact. Could such a heterogenous population live together peacefully amid all these factors; and could they demonstrate a community of equals working together on shared interests? Our faculty was a wonderful collection of mostly young adults with work experience in the Peace Corps and the relatively new federal domestic version of the Peace Corps., VISTA (Volunteers in Service to America). [As an aside- I would run into one of these counselors a year and a half later, during fall break of my first year of college. We bumped into each other in a bookstore across the street from the United Nations headquarters in New York. Who would have thought in July 1966, this kid from The Project would be in New York City a mere sixteen months later?] OK- consider a few memories from these six weeks before moving on to the senior year.

"Get out of bed you sleepy heads, there's a brand-new day ahead."That was our clarion call every morning from counselor James Elam. I never got tired of hearing that call. I am not and never have been an early morning riser. The nature of my existence has been such that I have often had to be up early. These six weeks were no exception. We were up early for breakfast as a group. We would get our daily briefing and be on our way to the day's schedule. Depending on the day and week, the plan might include lectures, small group discussion sessions, and field trips, either local or within 100 miles. One day a week, we went into the "hollers" to see what VISTA was doing in this poverty-stricken swath of Appalachian coal country. By now, you have been made aware of my deep-seated shyness. Finding myself immersed in these types of settings with 120 kids I did not know was hard. I was interested in the subject matter and the scope of the mission. I was uncomfortable at first and had a tough time reaching out and making friends. I liked my two roommates well enough. We got along fine. The Jewish kid from New York was the alpha male in the group, and the Black kid from Alabama was a lot like me in his shyness.

Nevertheless, we got along just fine when together in the room. We just didn't seek each other out to develop a friendship outside the confines of our shared sleeping quarters. That meant I had to make friends elsewhere. Fortunately, I was able to do that well enough. It had not occurred to me until sitting down to write this, but my two closest friends during this time turned out to be from the South. I don't remember that being intentional. I hadn't realized it until now, fifty-seven years later. I should not be surprised. The sociologist in me knows this is normal behavior. Those two friends, Bill Lindley from VA and Zylie Warren from GA, and I spent much of our free time together. Bill and I were alike in many ways; both shy and willing to gravitate to people and places where we felt safe. Zylie was a little less so, but still inclined to seek safe surroundings. None of us stayed in touch after the Encampment. I enjoyed those weeks together. In retrospect, I wish I had reached out to maintain those friendships. Failing to maintain friend relationships over time and wishing I had is one of my most heartbreaking realizations as I have grown older. I'll never know the joys, and perhaps some disappointments, I have missed by letting these casual friendships fade away so quickly after the physical proximity ended. I would make the same observation, even more profoundly, as it relates to my high school friends.

It became clear early on that a significant focus of the program would be related to race relations. I knew going in this would be the case. Still, I was a white male from the South who, by definition, was the villain in these conversations. It is not my intention in this epistle to relive those conversations now. The climate within which those discussion, sometimes arguments, occurred did precisely what the creators of the Encampment intended it to do. I know that Bill and I were the first white Southerners they had met for many of the kids there. There were others there as well. Likewise, I had never met anyone from outside North Carolina, other than the Air Force kids I knew at school. The bottom line is that my mindset was positively influenced and has had a lifelong impact. Some kids from New York, California, and other points north and west went home with a different view of at least some young folks from my part of the country. An example of what I am talking about came from one of our reading assignments. Among the many established (or, in some cases, new to the scene) writers I was exposed to was Eldridge Cleaver. We read about his activism and his angry, violent inclinations regarding "the movement." His book *Soul on Ice* had just been written but wouldn't be published until 1968. Reading about his story, and then three years later in college reading the book, I had to admit that I understood how he arrived at the place he was, given the road traveled to get there. I did not agree with the violent uprisings occurring in parts of the country. I could see something of the genesis from which they sprang. I grew up poor, living in The Project, in the South. I began to understand I had no clue what growing up poor and Black in the South was like. That realization began a lifelong effort to be consciously aware of that distinction. I don't know how successful I have been in that effort. I know I have tried to live and interact with life to be open to the reality of these differences and their influence on the decisions we all make and the paths we pursue.

One of the most impactful experiences relative to this revelation involved a girl from New York. Isabella Contreras was from East Harlem, better known then as Spanish Harlem. She was somewhat darker skinned with long black hair. She was absolutely stunning. It never occurred to me to be put off by her ethnicity; quite the contrary. I was smitten by her, as were any number of guys in the Encampment. As the weeks passed and we shared time in small group sessions, we formed a friendship. I had never known anyone who spoke Spanish as their first language. Remember, this was the mid-60s, and I lived in eastern North Carolina. Somewhere along the way, I learned something about Isabella that was not obvious from the start.

I knew she was of Hispanic background. I learned she was of mixed heritage. Her father was from Puerta Rico, and her mother was African American. When I first discovered this, I didn't know how to react. That information didn't alter in any way how I felt about Isabella. I was sixteen, an American male, and I had developed a real crush on her, something beyond friendship. She was very appealing in many ways. Even though I was shy and reserved in many social situations, we enjoyed each other's company. I'm sure she did not feel the same attraction to me as I did to her; hope always springs eternal, though. I began to wrestle with the juxtaposition of my feelings towards Isabella against what I had been taught all my life regarding Black folks. How could I possibly have the feelings I had for this beautiful girl from New York if what I had been told was true? It just didn't mesh. My "love" interests would be directed elsewhere as the weeks went on. I still wonder to what extent my willingness to allow those interests to shift focus was influenced by this knowledge. I don't know. I continued to see Isabella as a beautiful girl to whom I was attracted in many ways. I also know this question followed me home. Previously, I wrote about working in tobacco with Uncle Walter and Aunt Laulas and having lunch at their house. A wall began to crumble somewhere between my exposure to Eldridge Clever and my attraction to Isabella.

In addition to the social engagement being experienced on campus, we campers were introduced to the native inhabitants of this economically depressed heart of Appalachia. We would spend one full day in the communities each week, visiting locations of interest and significance. We would meet VISTA volunteers and other non-profit groups working to improve the lives of families caught in the never-ending spiral of poverty in those mountain "hollers." We participated in manual labor projects. We conducted door-to-door surveys. We lived one week in families' homes in the "hollers." (I would love to have been a fly on the wall when the VISTA staffers were asking for volunteers from families for this project.)

I spent a week with a family- a father, a mother, and two children. I met children who had never worn shoes during the summer and never owned a pair of new shoes. I slept on an old feather bed, much like the beds our ancestors might have had in their homes a hundred years ago. Our breakfast and supper consisted of meat and vegetables from the family's stock and garden and storage cellar. Water came from their well, and milk came from their cow-unprocessed by modern standards. This experience opened my eyes to a different level of poverty than the one I was living. For me, these days were informative. For some of my fellow campers, whose backgrounds were significantly more economically and socially advantaged, these day trips were more than eye-opening. They were transformative-at least for the time being. I have no way of knowing the long-term impact of their experiences. I can only imagine that many of those six-week friends found their lives changed in ways not unlike my life, which was changed by my exposure to Cleaver and Isabella.

During these six weeks, I met and conversed, socially or programmatically, with many of the 120 kids in the Encampment. I met kids from all socioeconomic backgrounds and ethnic heritages. I met kids from various religious backgrounds and perspectives, including self-avowed atheists and agnostics. I didn't meet any Quakers, members of the Religious Society of Friends. I heard a lot about them though. When I first heard Quakers mentioned, it was during a group session discussing the anti-war movement of the time. The speaker was from Philadelphia. While she was not a Quaker, she often spoke about the efforts of Quakers in her hometown. She also talked about their work in inner-city homeless and hunger programs. Others chimed in from time to time and referenced Quakers.

To my knowledge, I did not meet any Quakers during those six weeks. No one ever stepped forth to identify themselves as such. These comments piqued my interest. I knew a Quaker back home in Goldsboro. My friend, Bud Andrews, was a Quaker. I learned later that not only was he a Quaker, but he also came from a lengthy line of Quakers. His family was influential in Goldsboro's small but active Quaker community. I made it a point to seek Bud out once I got home to learn more about these Quakers. I had no idea the degree to which that decision would direct much of the rest of my life.

The six weeks of the Encampment ended, and I returned to Goldsboro full of excitement over what I had experienced the past six weeks; and full of anticipation of what was just around the corner. Football camp was just ahead, and a whole new school year. It felt good to be excited. Ahead was a year that would, at times, fill me with every reason to believe in the best and look forward to a great future; and at other times, would take me back to that place I knew too well; a place where there was no reason to believe in the best and no expectation of success, joy, or happiness. But, for the moment, I could only see today, and today looked good. The tomorrows would come soon and often enough.

August arrived and the Earthquakes were back to The Hill. Once again, work was hard, dirty, and sweaty, and life was GOOD! I had a new pair of managers working with me this year. Duffy Smith, a junior, was one of the many Air Force brats in our midst. Duffy was a serious golfer and one of the funniest guys around back then. He did a good job for us. And, he always could be counted on for a laugh. I didn't see Duffy after I graduated from high school. His Air Force father was transferred towards the end of the school year. Years later, I would reacquaint myself with Duffy quite by chance. After retirement, I worked part-time with RHINO Sports Entertainment Services, a customer services provider for college athletics and other large venue events. When I showed up for my first group training session, I was seated across the table from a man who looked a little familiar. During a break, this guy asked me if I knew a "Gene" Gurley. My name tag said "Anthony" Gurley. Anthony is my first name. As a child, I was known as "Gene," my middle name. It wasn't until my first real job as an adult that I had the nerve to go to "Anthony." I immediately recognized his name and put it together with a familiar face. We had a wonderful reunion and have continued to enjoy that reconnection. We both continue to work part-time for RHINO.

The other new manager was Charlie Watson. Charlie was another kid from The Project. He was two years behind me in school and had a connection with the head baseball coach at GHS, George Whitfield, who also assisted with football. Charlie was a good worker and a very funny guy. He would also go to work at Wilber's BBQ, making it a full-time job after high school. Like Duffy, we did not stay in touch after my graduation. However, we reconnected at the 50th reunion of the class of '67 football squad. What a joy to get back together. Since then, Charlie, who moved to Illinois some years ago and worked for Church's Chicken, has been back to North Carolina twice and stayed in my home both times. It has been one of the peaks in recent years to re-friend Charlie. His life has not been easy. It has been good for him to reconnect also.

The 1966 football team and season (graduating class of 1967) were memorable. The process and auxiliary events were much like the previous year. The additional year of experience and work, physical development, and other talent from new juniors and a couple of sophomores made us a team to be reckoned with. Early on, I followed up on my commitment to contact Bud about the Quakers. He invited me to come to meeting (church) with him one Sunday. By now, you may have noticed a glaring absence of anything about my church life, my faith walk. I attended church for as long as I can remember, until I was old enough to get a work permit and got the job at Wilber's.

Now, I was intent on looking at this Quaker thing. So, I accepted Bud's invitation. He agreed to drive me to Wilber's as soon as the meeting was over. Wilber agreed to my being about fifteen minutes late. I attended my first service at Goldsboro Friends Meeting in early September. I cannot tell you what the sermon was about. I did enjoy listening to the preacher. He and I would get to know each other well in years to come. What I enjoyed most about that first service was watching and listening (mostly watching) to the pianist playing the hymns the congregation sang. The pianist, Bailey Lowe, was Bud's cousin. I had seen her in passing at school. She was in our class. I had never actually spoken to her or even been close to her. We didn't share any classes. During that one hour on Sunday morning, all I could focus on was her. Suddenly, my interest in learning more about the Quaker church grew exponentially. I became a regular attendee, joining the church later that year. Bailey and I would go on to date some that year. She was my date to the athletic banquet/dance and the Jr-Sr Dance that following spring. It is awkward to write about this now. It is not too much of an exaggeration to say I was in love with Bailey. I was seventeen years old then. I understand what teenage crushes are, and I know all about the "puppy love" that can engulf an adolescent boy. That is not what I experienced. I have been happily married to Becky, the cute nurse farmer's daughter for fifty-one years now. But then, in 1966-67, I was in love, as real as any love has ever been. I wanted so much for Bailey to feel about me the way I felt about her. It was never to be. I enjoyed our time together and was painfully disappointed when she did not show a similar feeling. The school year ended, and Bailey left for college. I would see her only a few times after that. I stayed in touch with her parents when I returned to Goldsboro for family functions.

I would attend church at the Quaker meeting. Bailey's father and I got along well. I was never what her mother had in mind for her daughter. I often stopped by her parent's house to visit on those trips. When Bailey's father passed away, I attended his funeral. Bailey asked me to continue stopping by when I visited Goldsboro. Knowing I was checking in on her mom would mean a lot to her. I promised her I would. And I have done so. Bailey passed away in 2016 after a short illness. I continued to check in with her mom when I was in Goldsboro until her death a couple of years ago.

The running joke about that year at Goldsboro Friends Meeting and my introduction to Bailey has been that I started attending the meeting out of a genuine desire to know more about Quakerism. I continued to participate in the meeting out of another burning desire. As fate would have it, one desire would grow and guide many of my decisions for years to come. The other desire would fall victim to choices beyond my control. I have long since accepted that both developments were for the best. I remember having a conversation about this with my wife some years ago; probably not a good thing to do. It was awkward. I shared with her my feelings at the time and my continued affection for Mr. & Mrs. Lowe. I told her about my sitting in the car a block from Bailey's house one night after taking her home. I sat there crying to myself. I knew what I felt, and as much as I hated it, I knew she did not feel the same way. To my amazement, Becky said she understood. Not only did she understand, but she was also grateful for that time in my life and the role Bailey, and her family, played in it. Her rationale- the man she loved and had decided to spend the rest of her life with didn't just happen into existence. I was the physical, spiritual, intellectual, and emotional integration of all the parts up to that point. The time and life experiences I shared with Bailey and her family played no small role in that amalgamation. Becky loved all of me, and all of me was at least the total of those times and experiences, perhaps more.

For the most part, school was going well. I was still doing well academically, although I struggled with physics, which lowered my grade point average. That was OK. I was still in the top 5% of the class. I had been elected vice-president of the Varsity Club- the club that every athlete letterman belonged to. I was the first non-athlete to be selected as an officer in the club. Although not a player, I did letter in three sports. I was proud of that. I don't know whether there has been a non-athlete to hold such office since then. An interesting irony-Ken Nunn was the president of the club. Ken was a stud on the football team and played both ways. He would go on to play collegiately at Elon College. He also wrestled and played basketball. Ken and I did not travel in the same circles in high school, and our lives would go in separate directions after high school. We would see each other when we both attended class reunions. When working on plans for our football reunion, I discovered Ken had recently returned from a work trip to Israel with a Baptist men's group with which he was active. I was intrigued. I could not imagine the Ken Nunn I knew from high school being interested in going to Israel, and certainly not as part of a Baptist work trip. I inquired about it, and another fantastic door opened. For now, it was just another old friend relationship rejoined, and a conscious realization of many years of memories not to be experienced and, therefore, not available to be missed.

With the end of football season came the onset of wrestling. More importantly, the season for college applications was in full swing. This was something alien to anything I had ever known.

On the college application scene, I knew I was looking at three schools- East Carolina, Catawba, and Guilford. There was a strong Catawba connection with our coaching staff. Ken Nunn, Mike DeGrechie, Ron Tingen, and I visited there. The three of them were being looked at for football, and I had an opportunity to be a manager/trainer for the football team. Guilford College in Greensboro was a possibility. The Quakers founded the college in 1837, and it still had a substantial Friends connection. Bud was going there, and I thought that might be a good fit. I liked the notion of going to a smaller school. East Carolina was in the mix as well. East Carolina Teachers College (it became East Carolina University- ECU in 1967) was where several of the coaches had done their graduate work. Coach Whisenhunt was a good friend of Coach Clarence Stasavich, the head coach at ECU. Coach Whis had talked to Coach Stas about me, and I could receive a partial scholarship there as a manager/trainer on their football team. Coach Whis offered to take me to Greenville to meet Coach Stas and tour the school. We never got there though. The school car we were taking broke down a couple of miles outside Goldsboro. We never rescheduled the trip. So, I had options. I was confident I would get into each of these schools. And I did.

After the state wrestling championships in the spring, I had to decide what I would do for the rest of the school year. I had never enjoyed working with the track program. I didn't want to do that anymore. I did not want to let Coach Whis down. Somehow I managed to get the courage to tell him I wanted not to do track this year. I wanted to see if Coach Whitfield would be interested in having me as a team manager and trainer for baseball. The two of them agreed this would be OK. For me, it was fantastic. I loved baseball and always have. I wished many times I had tried to play while in school. By then, just being a part of the team in that capacity was enough. Early on, I experienced a real serendipity. Someone told Coach Whitfield I had been a good catcher in Little League; I suspect it was the starting catcher. In addition to performing the duties of manager and trainer, I took on the role of batting practice catcher on practice days. I loved it. There was no glory in it. I didn't dress out on game days. That would come later. But I was in a place I loved to be. And I was contributing in a tangible way. My catching batting practice saved the starter from having to do so. It prevented him from getting unnecessarily hurt in practice and reduced his fatigue between game days. Later, as the season progressed, I was allowed to dress out on game days. I would warm up relief pitchers.

I got into one game as a pinch runner. I was dumbfounded. I had yet to learn what the signals from the coach were for bunt, or steal, or whatever. I remember Ron Tingen being the first base coach and giving me a hard time about it. He had a fun time tricking and teasing me while I was on first base. For better or for worse, the next batter struck out, and I was left on first. That's probably a good thing. I have no idea what would have happened had I had to run the bases. It had been over three years since I had done that in a real game. Those were good times. We had a decent team. More importantly, we had a brotherhood.

During that time of the year, as seniors were winding down and post-graduation plans were taking shape, various scholarship programs and other awards were announced. I garnered my share of attention. Each year the Goldsboro Optimist Club conducted an oratorical contest. They set a topic and invited high school senior boys to write a speech and give it before a live panel of judges. Coach Whisenhunt, an active participant in the club, suggested I should apply. I was reluctant to do so. I was thrilled he thought I could do it. I don't remember the topic. I do remember I entered and made the first cut.

Three of us were selected to give our speeches, without notes, before the full Optimist Club. First, second, and third place prizes would be awarded- trophies and small scholarship awards. I was up against a friend who was to go to Wake Forest University and become a highly successful attorney. The other candidate was one of the many air force kids in our class. At the end of the program that night, I took home the top trophy and scholarship prize. I was on top of the world. At the time, I didn't know whether I won because I really did outperform the other contestants. Or, did I win because I did OK, reasonably on par with the other two, and I had the most significant financial need by far? I'll never know. I'm not sure it would have mattered had I known. Years later, when I reflected on this event and the subsequent professional lives of the three of us, I would find myself going to that place again. I would compare my career and financial accomplishments to Warren and Lester and come to one conclusion. What a significant underachiever I have been. It's too late to do anything about it. I must live with the consequences- or do I?

The name that was noticeably missing from the competition was Danny Davis. I don't know why Danny didn't compete in this event. He would have been a formidable opponent. We would share a competition that spring. Danny and I were two of six GHS candidates for the prestigious Morehead Scholarship at UNC. The Morehead was then, and still is, one of the most prestigious undergraduate scholarship programs at any university in the country. It was a full ride, room, board, tuition, and fees. I was surprised when the local nominating committee nominated me.

When I saw who the other candidates were, I knew I could not win. But I was honored to be there. After my interview, I knew for sure I would not win. It was the worst I have ever performed in a live interview. There were five or six people on the interviewing committee. I didn't know any of them. But when they introduced themselves, I knew their names. Everyone was either a doctor, a lawyer, a state politician, a judge, or a wealthy business owner, and all were distinguished UNC alums. After we completed the interviews and Danny was announced as the winner some days later, I was disappointed, but not surprised. And I must confess, Danny was the right choice. He did have all the credentials and fit the profile, a skill set and profile I would never possess.

One other student award program in the spring was the Senior Superlatives. Seniors voted on their classmates to be recognized in several categories, one male and one female-Most Popular, Most Friendly, Most Likely to Succeed, Most Intellectual, Best Personality, etc. There were a dozen or so of these things. Well, guess what? I was voted Best Personality for the male half of the team. I was astonished. I had no expectation of getting selected for anything. For years I looked back on that honor and was so proud. That really was one of those "peak" moments that years later morphed into another never-ending "valley." It was some years later that I realized what Best Personality really meant. High school students don't think in these terms. I don't think my classmates intentionally meant to insult me or Ashley. No! How did I come across to my classmates as the male member of our class with the Best Personality? Here's how. Always give in to someone else's position. Never raise a stink. Always be willing to take the back row or the second seat. Never seek to draw attention to self for recognition or achievement. Always smile and look friendly. That described me then, and for most of my life- not much of a blueprint for success, but a foolproof plan for being well-liked, at least on the surface.

My exposure to the Quaker church was parallel to what was going on in school during this year. My interest was genuinely tweaked during my time at the Encampment. I was curious after coming home and beginning my attendance at Goldsboro Friends Meeting. The pastor at the meeting was Willie Frye. Willie was married with three children. He was in his mid-thirties, and both looked and seemed young. He took an interest in me and made me feel very welcome, as did members of the meeting in general. Unfortunately, I would only be in meeting regularly for a year as I was heading off to college next fall. During the year, however, I developed friendships with older members of the church that would last for decades. The only members of the meeting who were my age that I continued to stay in touch with were my good friends Bud and Bill Scott. Bill would come to work at Guilford a couple of years after I did, heading up the grounds department. When I started attending the meeting, I had no idea I would become a member, becoming what the Quakers call a "convinced Friend." A "convinced Friend" is one who was not born into a Quaker family; one who, through association and shared experience, chooses to join in membership. A person born into a Quaker family, such as Bud, is known as a "birthright Friend."

A decision totally outside my realm of responsibility would prove to be life-altering for me. During the spring, Willie Frye was offered the pastor position at Winston-Salem Friends

Meeting. This was a promotion for Willie. Winston-Salem was
a much bigger city than Goldsboro, located in the Piedmont
Triad of North Carolina- Greensboro, Winston-Salem, and
High Point. The meeting there was much bigger as well. It was
a no-brainer for Willie and his family. When Willie accepted
the appointment, the Goldsboro meeting had to search for
his replacement. It was evident the meeting would not have a
replacement for Willie by the time he left. I'll always remember
the day Willie asked me to come by his office. He had something he wanted to talk to me about. As was, and still is, my
nature, I was petrified. What had I done? Well, I hadn't done
anything other than catch the eye of Pastor Frye. He sensed I
was taking my exploration of Quakerism seriously and was on
a path that might lead to a call to full-time ministry. I hadn't
thought much about that but was willing to consider it. Willie
had heard about my winning the Optimist Oratorical Contest.
It had been in the local newspaper, the Goldsboro News-Argus.
Bud might have told him. Maybe Ms. Ina Mixon, a senior
member of the meeting and an algebra teacher at school, had
mentioned it.

Anyway, Willie asked if I would be interested in "filling the
pulpit" after his departure for the remainder of the summer
until it was time for me to head off to Guilford College. I would
not be expected to perform any non-preaching duties of the
pastor. Those duties, mostly hospital visits, would be assumed
by members of the meeting. I would be paid a fair salary for the
weeks I worked. I would use the pastor's office and library to
help prepare sermons. I didn't have to think about it. I said "yes"
at once. I was always confident speaking in front of a crowd. I
hate having to schmoose at social functions. I have rarely been

ill at ease in front of a crowd, assuming I know something about the subject matter I am addressing.

I would end up preaching a total of eight Sundays. For the most part, I knew enough about the subject matter, and I was creative enough to use tools to get through it well enough. By summer's end, I was ready to head to Greensboro, and Goldsboro Friends Meeting was prepared to greet its new full-time pastor. That experience did, as Willie suggested, start me thinking perhaps a call to the ministry in the Quaker church might be in my future.

I would be remiss if I failed to offer a final thought about this last year in high school. As noted, the year was a record year in terms of athletic achievements for the Earthquakes. None of us had any notion of how exceptional and unusual those years were. Now, fifty-five years have passed, and both our class and members of that football team (including juniors and sophomores) have stayed in touch. Today I still think about the Saturday nights I would sit at home, without a date, with no money or car, feeling sorry for myself. I remember sitting on the front porch, moving back and forth in that old green aluminum glider, imagining what certain classmates were doing while I was sitting at home. I remember crying my eyes out, wishing for something that would never be.

No matter how many wins our teams had, or how much acclaim I received, none of that could overcome my sense of being on the outside looking in. That sense would follow me for years. Today, as I write this in my home office, my son's converted bedroom, I still am overpowered by those feelings. I have tried all my adult life to walk in the faith I was introduced to at an early age. Yet, that tugging at my heart has always been there. I have always known or wanted to believe that there is a power more significant than the circumstances of the moment. Which is it- have I always *known* it, or have I merely wanted to *believe* it? I don't know. There is a difference. In those moments when I find myself on the outside looking in, I am reduced to wanting to *believe*. When the best of life is going on, and I am experiencing all its fullness, then I *know*. Such was, and is, the dilemma.

Time moves on. My days at Goldsboro High School came to an end. Greensboro, Guilford College, and life after Goldsboro lay just ahead.

Wow! Talking about therapeutic and cathartic, all at the same time. This chapter looked at such a small window of time. I could write a whole manuscript about those couple of years. The peaks- the valleys- the noise, the rah-rahs, the exuberance-; the quiet- the stillness- the tears- the anger- the utter desire to stop feeling this way. This has been hard. Too many times the emotions get jump-started, only to be smothered. Life had had way too many of these repeating episodes- different storylines, repeating plots. Life seems to be that way.

Reliving those years has prompted yet another review of the storyboard, more inquiring into the "what ifs" in life. We all experience them, the "what ifs." What if I had won the Morehead? Would I have dropped out or flunked out of Carolina in two years? Or, would I have cruised right through and gone to law school or gotten an MBA, and who knows what? How different might my life have been? How much more traveling and enjoying this remarkable creation we call Earth? Oh, how I would love to know what that life would look like today. But then, the beautiful things and people I love about my actual path might not have materialized. How does one assess what might have been compared to what was and is? How does one escape this never-ending search for such peace? Too much focus on the "what ifs" will drive one mad.

How does one present oneself so that his/her classmates see them as a Best Personality superlative, while also carrying inwardly all this "stuff"? Or are the two mutually exclusive? This is complicated. I once heard the expression, "Ignorance is bliss." Maybe it is. Becky and I joke about whether I am curious or inquisitive. I mentioned once I was not curious about anything. I would never have made a good lawyer- not nearly curious enough. Becky responded that I am one of the most curious people she has ever known. I don't know. I won't argue the point. I can only imagine how less stressful and much happier life would be if I could just let it go and not reflect so on past failures, disappointments, and shortcomings.

When I was in high school, I had no idea what a grand time I was living in. I lived too much in the valleys and could not see and commit to my innermost recesses those peaks I encountered frequently. I couldn't do it. I can't seem to do it now. What else is left?

Chapter 8

FIRST TRY AT COLLEGE

AUGUST 1967 ARRIVED after a busy summer of working in tobacco and Wilber's, preaching at the Quaker meeting, and getting ready for college. I would be the first in my family to do that. My nearest sibling, Faye, went to business school in Raleigh. I would be the first to go away for a four-year degree and live that American Dream of college life. Looking back now, I had no idea what lay ahead. I was so ill-prepared for it. I have often suggested I might have been much better off had I gone to work for a year or two before college. Maybe then I would have been more mature and better prepared for the academic and social rigors I would encounter. That option, however, was never considered. What if? After all, I had been a stellar student and visible leader in many ways. Once the notion of going to college solidified into a real mission along the path between junior high school and high school, I never even thought of not going. Once I decided to attend college, I never imagined not getting into a good one. Finally, once in, failing or dropping out never entered my mind. To do so would have constituted such an embarrassment I could not fathom it. At first, my lofty expectations of Greensboro were right on track and clearly within reach. I'm not sure when it happened; or how it happened. I am sure there were multiple causes.

Somewhere towards the end of my first year, or early in the second, I began to sow the seeds of my academic freefall at Guilford. Two years after I arrived at Quaker-Tech (not a real name for Guilford, but one some of us liked to throw around occasionally), I would find myself saying goodbye. I did not know whether I would ever return or whether I would ever enroll in college again anywhere. Both Guilford and I shared in the decision for me to leave the college. Had I not withdrawn, I would have been dismissed academically. I'm not proud of that. I never told my mother. She never knew anything about my academic struggles that second year. All she knew was I had decided to take two years off and work in a hospital in Winston-Salem to fulfill my military obligation.

I arrived in the parking lot of the "Quacker Box," the old gymnasium on the east side of the central part of the campus, next door to the baseball field. The football field sat just south of the baseball field. Joyce and my mama drove me to Greensboro that day. I was going to be a manager for the football team and train to work as a trainer as well. As such, I had to arrive early, before other first-year students. The football team arrived early, and the managing and training staff had to be there before they came. Harmon Keller, a Junior, and the Head Trainer welcomed me. I was one of two freshmen joining the staff. Harmon was a Quaker also, a birthright Friend. Joyce and Mama didn't stay long. We drove through the main campus drive before arriving at the gym parking lot.

Once there, I removed my valued worldly possessions: one big suitcase, a footlocker, a gym bag, and a cardboard box about the size of medium size microwave. Everything I owned that was worth anything materially or sentimentally was in those containers. We stopped for lunch along the way, so we didn't need to eat when we got there. We unloaded the car, and I gave Mama and Joyce hugs. Just as unceremonially as we had arrived, they were returning to Goldsboro. In those days, it was about a three and half-hour drive from Goldsboro to Guilford College, driving through Smithfield, Raleigh, and Durham rather than bypassing them, mainly on a two-lane road until past Durham. Nowadays, the trip is about two and a quarter hours, with all of it on four-lane interstate highways and bypassing Smithfield, Raleigh, and Durham altogether. I connected with Harmon, who introduced me to the head coach, and a couple of assistant coaches. I was at college and ready to go. I was, at one time, both excited and frightened.

It would be two weeks before other non-football first-year students would arrive, followed by other returning students in three days. These first two weeks were full of football. In some ways, it reminded me of our Earthquakes camps. Two-a-day practices with skull sessions at night were the norm. We stayed in a barracks-type locker room in the basement of the gym. We could only move into our dorm rooms once the other students arrived. The role of the managers was like what it had been in high school.

On the other hand, the trainer's job was quite different-mainly in the scale of the job. Far more players used the services of the trainer(s) at Guilford than had been my experience in high school. I was comfortable with that. It meant I could move in that direction more quickly than expected. Harmon needed more help. He was eager to train and bring me along to assist. The number of players on the team was more than in high school. More players with knee braces and more backs and receivers required pre-practice and pre-game ankle taping. We had more players needing post-practice and post-game heat or ice treatments. I loved it. Guilford played in the National Association of Intercollegiate Athletics (NAIA), an association of small colleges and universities. In that context, Guilford had a surprisingly good program. I was excited to be a part of it. These two weeks of pre-season practice passed quickly. The upper-level students were good about welcoming us first-year students. Several first-year students were going to be real contributors. One of those freshmen was Jay White. He and I discovered we had dated the same girl in high school. My date at the Varsity Club dance in my sophomore year was Rita Howell. She had moved to Jay's hometown before our junior year. There she met Jay, and they dated regularly through much of high school. Jay would have a successful career as a high school coach in North Carolina.

We could move into our dorms when the other new students arrived for first-year orientation. I moved into a ground-floor room in the Center Section of Cox Hall. Cox Hall was one of the older dorms on campus. It was designed in five sections of three floors, with four rooms on each floor housing two students each. A communal bathroom was at the rear of each floor in each section. The building was old. The heating system was unreliable. The floor creaked, and the walls were porous. We loved it. It was the most fun men's dorm on campus. I had already moved in when my roommate arrived. Winston Puckett was a big kid, probably three or four inches taller than me and fifty pounds heavier. He was from Winston-Salem. He was a Moravian, a religious sect I had never heard of and knew nothing about; one that, as I learned later, was instrumental in the founding of the village that would become the city of Winston-Salem. It is still a significant presence in the city, including Salem Academy & College dating back to 1772. Winston planned to go into the ministry and, indeed, would go on to the Moravian Seminary in Bethlehem, PA.

Winston and I would room together our first two years. He and I were different; everything from our family and economic backgrounds to our tastes in music. Like me, Winston had several friends from high school who were also new freshmen at Guilford. Back in those days, Guilford attracted a good cadre from Goldsboro. Four of us from GHS arrived at Guilford that fall. There were several more already there in the upper classes. Several classmates joined Winston from Winston-Salem. I would get to know them as casual friends. My introduction to alcohol, which was short-lived, can be attributed to Winston and his high school friends.

I thoroughly enjoyed my first year at Guilford and did well in the classroom and elsewhere. The football was good. As is usually the case, first-year students are at the bottom of the team ladder, and I knew that. Harmon did an excellent job of welcoming Weldon and me into the fold and nurturing us along the way. Much like my high school experience with sports, I was going places I had never been before, this time into South Carolina and Virginia. We closed the season with a 6-4 record and two small college All-Americans on the squad. Looking back at the list of opponents compared to the college's current competition is revealing. Back then, Guilford competed primarily against schools affiliated with the NAIA. These were small colleges that awarded athletic grants. Every college on the schedule during my first year that was then an NAIA school is now an NCAA school, either D-1 or D-2. Guilford transitioned from its NAIA affiliation to the NCAA D-111 in the mid-1980s. D-111 is a non-scholarship division. I was the Director of Financial Aid at the time of the transition. It is safe to say the overall athletic talent level turned downward. Whether the move was good for the college or not, I don't know. I enjoyed my time with the football team.

While football was in season, there was the matter of classes and schoolwork to settle into. Before arriving on campus, I decided I would be a biology major. That was a stretch for me. I had done well in biology in high school but had yet to take advanced-level courses. I wanted to be a professional athletic trainer. I loved my experience in high school and was good at it. There were only a few professional trainers around. I had a sense that it was a profession on the rise. My goal was to get a job at a college or university. Biology would be an excellent undergraduate major for that path. It would be a good major also should I go on to graduate school in physical therapy.

When I put together my fall class schedule with the help of a faculty advisor, I signed up for a General Biology class with a lab. Guilford had a two-semester foreign language requirement, so I scheduled German 101. I filled the rest of the schedule with a math requirement, an English Composition, and an elective- Personal & Community Hygiene. That didn't look like too much to start. Cliff Rogers taught the German class. He was a man whom I would get to know well over the years. He became a good friend and mentor. The English Composition course was a hoot. Heather Del Aqua was the instructor. She was somewhat young and new to the job.

I had been a solid A student in high school. I knew college would be different. I was sure I could hold my own. And hold my own, I did, with one exception. That exception was in the field where I could not falter if I was serious about my career path. By the time I was halfway through the semester, I realized I would fail my biology class. I had never failed a class in my life. I had rarely made anything below a high B throughout my entire junior high and senior high years. Failing a class, particularly one on which my entire career path plan rested, was unimaginable. But failing, I was. What I discovered has bothered me to this day. I could read the textbook and understand it. It was hard. I could memorize the things I needed to remember. What I couldn't do was look into a microscope and have any understanding of what I was seeing. I tried! I've never been good at asking for help. By the time it became clear to me and the professor I was not getting it, it was too late to salvage the term. I still don't know what the issue was. Was I not trying hard enough? Was I not focusing somehow? Was there an underlying physiological condition that caused this visual disconnect? I don't know. All I know is that my plan to major in biology and be a professional athletic trainer came to a halt early in my college career. I'll never know whether there might have been another solution to my problem. A different option might have surfaced if I had been more forceful in seeking a resolution or asking for help. But I wasn't, and one didn't. Like everything else, the semester moved on anyway, and I had to roll with it. Giving up on the plan I wanted to pursue, I signed up for a spring schedule that did not include any biology classes. I quit, an option I would default to way too often in the coming years. I would have to find a different path. I needed to think about it. I just took a vanilla schedule in the spring. I just wanted to get through.

One of the real serendipities of the first year at Guilford took place after football season. Guilford did not have a wrestling team, so I did not have a winter sports team to work for as I did in high school. Guilford had an outstanding, national-caliber basketball team. They already had their trainer though. Remember, Guilford participated in the NAIA. These were smaller schools you didn't see playing on television. There was some outstanding talent playing in those schools across the country. The breadth of basketball talent distributed among the NCAA Div. 1 schools today did not exist in the 60s. Only 23 teams made the NCAA national tournament, and only a handful of colleges competed at that level. Outside the NCAA process, there was the NAIA. Guilford was one of those schools that had developed a high level of play, attracting players who did not get into or were not recruited by the Big Boys.

The head coach at Guilford was Jerry Steele. His assistant was Jack Jensen. Both were Wake Forest graduates who played for the famous Wake coach Bones McKinney. Together, they built a strong program at Guilford. Some folks "in the know" in those days would argue the team that took the floor for the Quakers in the fall of 1967 may have been one of the two best teams in North Carolina. The team, led by 6'8' center Bob Kaufman from The Bronx, would have a 21-3 season that winter and win both conference and district championships, losing only three games all year. Bob would be the third player drafted in that year's NBA draft, behind future Hall of Famers Elgin Baylor and Wes Unseld. (Players from schools like Guilford rarely made it to the NBA, much less get drafted high in the first round.) It was a season to remember. They went to Kansas City for the national tournament, ranked #1 in the country in the NAIA, and seeded #1 in the tournament. The campus was afire with enthusiasm. Every day in the caf leading up to the tournament, students were greeted with a loud repeating rendition of the "Kansas City" song by Fats Domino. It was a 'happenin' place, right up until the team's first game in the tournament. The year to be remembered came to a sudden and unforeseen end. Oshkosh St. upset the mighty Quakers in the opening round. Seldom have my emotions gone from such a high level of exuberance to such a devastating low level of disappointment in such a moment.

I told you I had no team to work for during the winter season. That was new for me; the first time I had been in that boat since before junior high school. It did not last long. I don't know if it resulted from a bet or a dare. Or, did someone reach out and make an offer Walter Harris and I could not refuse? At any rate, Walter Harris, another first-year from Oak Ridge, TN, and I became the first two male cheerleaders in the history of Guilford College. At least, that is our story, and we are sticking to it. We could find no record of any male cheerleaders in any yearbooks before us. Walter and I became friends early in the semester. By stature, he was a bit shorter than me. Neither Walter nor I made the grade by today's male cheerleader standards. Neither of us could do the kinds of acrobatic and gymnastic stunts you see these guys do today. Somehow though, there we were. We were full of spirit and energy. We did work hard and managed to do a couple of stunts. My partner, Ould run to me from a few yards away. Just before reaching me, she would take a flying leap with arms outstretched. My job was to catch her, placing my hands firmly at the center of her hips. With some work and a lot of trust we got to be good at this. The other stunt involved even more faith on my partner's part. She would jump into my arms, me holding her with my right arm and hand under her back and shoulders. My left arm and hand cradled her beneath her knees. On signal, I would swing her to my right. Letting go of her legs and wrapping her body around my back. I would almost immediately let go of her upper body with my right arm and, with all my might, swing her as aggressively as I could back up around my back with my left arm and upper body, catching her upper body to end up back in the original cradle in the arms position. She not only had to have complete trust in me, but she also had to have enormous strength and body control to avoid striking her head and getting her upper body up to where I could catch her. She was amazing!

That season, and my time as a cheerleader, is one of the best memories of my first two years at Guilford. The summer after that year, we went to Hattiesburg, MS, to the University of Southern Mississippi campus for a week-long college cheerleader camp. We rode the train to get there. I was having the time of my life. How many college guys would give anything to be in my shoes; it makes one ask the question- why had there not been any male cheerleaders before? I don't know. All I know is Walter and I were living a dream.

The remainder of the semester moved along. Classes were OK, except for biology. I should have dropped it earlier and perhaps avoided an 'F." I didn't. When the semester ended, I went home to The Project and Mama. I had only been gone four months. I had changed. I had no idea what the next few months or years would hold. I could not imagine the events I would experience over the next eighteen months, the next three and a half years, and so on. What I did know, even though I could not articulate it then, was that I had changed. I knew I would never go home to live again. I was sure I would never return to Goldsboro to live and work again.

The rest of that first year at Guilford proved to carry the seeds of my undoing- at least for the near term. I was a poor kid from The Project who was a good student. I was also terribly shy, introverted, and ashamed of my origins. I had always done exceptionally well in school. Now, a freshman in college, I was not "getting it." I began to doubt if I could make it. The remainder of the year became a maze of distractions, and disappointments, with the occasional mixture of aha moments. My good friend from high school, Bud Andrews, was there. He and I would continue to be good friends, but we didn't spend much time together. As I write this, Bud and I are in our 70s. We live 100 miles apart, and our lives have taken very different paths. Each of us still thinks of the other as his best friend in life.

Previously, when talking about my experience with the Encampment for Citizenship, I mentioned that I would run into one of the staffers a couple of years later in New York. Well, I did. When Fall Break was just a few weeks off, Winston, my roommate, asked me if I was interested in going to New York during the Break. You cannot imagine my disbelief. My only experience traveling outside North Carolina was my summer Encampment in Barbourville. I spent six weeks in the heart of coal country, eating, working, playing, and thinking with 120 kids from every corner and ethnic background in the country. A year later, I was living with around a thousand students, mostly from up and down the east coast and some of the Midwest. My horizons had grown by leaps and bounds during that period of time. I had never given any thought to going to New York. From my starting point, that might have been another country. And going to another country was never going to happen. (Or would it?) I had heard about Guilford's study abroad program, some short-term off-campus trips during Fall and Spring Breaks, and a summer offering. I asked Winston what he was talking about; why New York, and what would we do there?

Winston explained the deal and brought me an information flyer about the trip.

A geology professor would be the faculty leader. We would take a bus to and from New York and stay in a YMCA with low-cost bed and bath facilities for visiting college study groups. We would visit museums, go to a couple of Broadway shows, tour the United Nations Headquarters, and see the city's sites. We would ride the subway and see the Statue of Liberty. I was sold. I wanted so badly to go. I knew several of the students who were going. I knew we would have a great time. Oh, and yes! It would be a legitimate educational experience!

Those few days had a profound effect. It wasn't so much what we saw in the museums or the plays. (We saw "Man of La Mancha" and "MacBird!") I became a great fan of "Man of La Mancha." As I write this, I can see three pairs of Don Quixote and Sancho Panza I have collected over the years from my wife's mission travels abroad. I had never had any alcohol before that trip. Winston had been to New York before and knew his way around. He and I went for a walk one evening and found ourselves at the skating rink at Rockefeller Center. We decided to sit and watch the skaters for a while. He suggested we order something to drink. I had no clue. He talked me into ordering a Whiskey Sour. I didn't know what was in it. I still don't know. But it was good, and I enjoyed it. That was the only alcohol I had on that trip. Winston and his friends from Winston-Salem would remedy that before too long back in North Carolina.

One of the evenings in the city before we went to the theatre, several of us went to dinner with the professor. It was one of those small, hole-in-the-wall local-favorite Italian restaurants, a place where you could get authentic Italian cuisine. There were about a dozen of us. I knew almost everybody. It was calming to discover I was not the only person for whom this was their first trip to New York. We enjoyed dinner and a fun time together, discussing our day's exploits. When we finished, and it was time to walk the few blocks to the theatre, we all settled the bill, giving our money to the Prof. He would pay the total bill as one, rather than the cashier having to settle it with one customer at a time. I did not have much experience dining out, certainly, in places like this. It certainly made sense to me to do it this way. It was a busy place and crowded. We were elbow to elbow in the crowd. So, we all got up and walked out front to clear some space. Dale gave our waiter the check and sufficient cash to cover the bill. A few minutes later, Dale joined us, and we were off to Broadway. Then suddenly, out of nowhere, we were (Dale was) accosted by a young man in black pants and a white shirt and black tie. He wore a small, folded white apron around his waist.

There was a moment of shock. Being the kid from The Project, I had seen television news and heard about the kinds of robberies and muggings people encountered on the streets of Big Cities. My first reaction was we were in the middle of such an encounter. Then, as suddenly as it came upon us, it became clear what was happening. What was happening, though not a robbery or mugging, was, to me, just as scary. The young man we all now recognized had come to collect his tip. Dale had walked out without leaving the expected (back then) 10% TIP. Dale was embarrassed. The young man was belligerent. The waiter made it clear he had been stiffed, and that would not do. Dale apologized profusely and assured the waiter it was an oversight. Dale gave him the TIP, and we were on our way. The waiter marched away, back to the restaurant, using language I had rarely heard outside a locker room brawl.

After the play, we returned to the Y. I'm sure some of our group snuck back out after curfew. Neither Winston nor I were among them. But my exciting day was not yet over. After returning to our room, I was not sleepy, so I decided to go downstairs to the basement pool and pool-lounge area. It was late, and I was the only person there. Shortly after I sat down to ponder the day and think about all I was experiencing, I had a visitor. She was another first-year student from New Jersey. I met her at the beginning of the trip. She was not someone I knew from campus. It was a little awkward. But I invited her to stay.

I guess I was as naïve as a just-turned-eighteen-year-old college guy could be. It quickly became apparent that Linda had not accidentally come to the basement pool to talk. She had called our room to speak with me, and Winston told her where I was. I had dated some in high school and "been in love." Since my arrival at Guilford, I had not dated much. I had been out with groups. I went to parties. I had not gone on a one-to-one date. Remember, I had no money or car and didn't drink. Frankly, Linda would not have been my choice for such if I had. She was nice enough and smart. I was not physically attracted to her in any way. She was not interested in discussing "MacBird!", the waiter, or anything else. I was in a place I had never been before. I was still a virgin, not because I wanted to be, but because no one I wanted to take that step with had ever allowed me to do so. I don't know how I would have reacted had any of those opportunities presented. I wasn't interested that night in that basement pool with that girl from NJ. For some time after that night, when back on campus and reliving the trip, I rethought that encounter and wondered what might have been different. I've retold this encounter because it serves as an example of many encounters in my life that I have relived and wondered 'What if." I have no regrets about saying 'No" to Linda. I do have regrets. There are numerous moments, encounters, and missed opportunities I regret I let get away. I am sure some would have proven to be wonderful open doors for achievement, advancement, or just plain old feel-good moments. Some, I am sure, would have led to the next failure, the next loss, the next missed opportunity. The question becomes: how does one know which outcome will follow? I do not regret my response to Linda. How do I know the result would not have been one I would have been happy to have experienced? I don't know. Much of my life has been subject to this confrontation. I have always tended to be slow to decide, stand back from uncertain outcomes, and second-guess myself, all of which are a guaranteed road to mediocrity and underachievement. No matter how wonderful the moment is or how vibrant the feeling is, there is always that place that lures me back. I have never felt so good or happy about any circumstance that I did not eventually fall back to that place. When our bus arrived back in Greensboro, I was already bemoaning that I "chickened out."."

So- we're back at Guilford and Fall Break is over. When the bus pulled onto the campus, I was so glad I had gone. When I got to my dorm room and got ready for bed, I found a nickel and four pennies in my pocket. So that's what I came home from a four-day trip to New York with- 9 cents. I was tickled to death. One of my favorite memories of Bud during this period, and one of those "aha" times, was our first-year English class. It was a writing class, taught by Heather Del Aqua. (Years later, I would get to know Heather on a professional level when I went to work at Guilford and she was still on the faculty there.) We didn't realize it was Heather's first year teaching at the college. Bud and I both loved her class and her. She was not right out of grad school but inexperienced as a classroom English teacher. She had yet to learn some of the tricks employed by more seasoned teachers to get a class to engage. Again, it was a creative writing class, and Heather was having difficulty engaging the class in discussion. She would present an idea or propose a scenario or plot and try to get the class to react. We had a class devoid of curiosity or imagination, or kids weren't awake yet. It was a mid-morning class.

I don't remember whose idea it was. Bud and I decided we could jump-start the class. We didn't tell Heather what we were going to do. Instead, we began responding vigorously to her pleas. It didn't matter what the subject was. Bud or I would react, and the other would immediately take an opposing position or point of view. Usually, after a few minutes of the two of us going after each other, Heather would real us back in, or others in the class would begin to jump in and carry the ball. That was, after all, the goal. We succeeded well in our plan and had great fun doing it. I'll remember a conversation in my office at the college some years after I started working there. By this time, Heather was up in years and near retirement. I had never told her my and Bud's scheme. That day something led me to bring it up. I told her about our intentional plan and how much fun we had. Heather had no idea. She had no idea it was all a ruse on our part, that we were playing off one another, that the positions we argued were not ours, but were required for the scheme to unfold. When I told her of our plot, she was immediately beside herself. We both nearly cried we laughed so hard.

Heather passed away not many years after that conversation. She is one of those memories from my first years at

Guilford that feels good as I sit writing. Other memories don't feel quite so good.

During the spring semester, I began to experience academic failure as I had never known before. Remember, I had been an athletic trainer in high school. I went to college with every expectation of pursuing an academic path that would prepare me to be a professional athletic trainer- and that was in the late 60s- long before the profession had become as prevalent as it is today. I was unprepared for the utter failure I experienced in my first biology class with a lab. I had never encountered failure like that before. However, that did not seal my academic fate and forever altered my career path. No- the failure was that the shy/introverted little boy in me would not reach out and ask for help. Not once did I seek help from the professor. Not once did I stop by his office and confess. No- I just went to class and tried to hide. I did the best I could on classwork and reading the textbook. I could not do the lab work. I have no memory of ever speaking with the instructor about this. I don't know whether he tried to reach me and offer help outside class or lab time. It doesn't matter. I needed help to see if I could "get there." I didn't get any help. It was my responsibility to ask for it. Once again, that lesson I learned at home early in life- don't ask for a damn thing- was overpowering rational thought.

At the same time, I was beginning to struggle even more with schoolwork. I was making some not-so-good choices outside the classroom. My roommate had several high school friends who were also at Guilford. He also had a couple of pals at Chapel Hill. I had never been around drinking much. No one in my family drank, to my knowledge. My good friend, Glenn Aycock, would drink some on weekends when we would go out. Frankly, he was the first person I ever saw drunk. He was a nasty drunk too. Other than that, I had lived a sheltered life regarding alcohol. The only time I had ever had any alcohol was after I arrived at Guilford and went on the fall break trip to New York I wrote about earlier. My whiskey sour with Winston at Rockefeller Center was all the alcohol I had on that trip or the rest of the fall semester. The spring semester came, and Chapel Hill called. Before I knew it, on a Saturday afternoon in February, Winston and I and a couple of his high school friends were off to visit other friends at Carolina.

The content of that trip is not important for this treatment, with one exception. We arrived on Franklin Street in time to pick up some sandals Winston and I had bought a few weeks earlier on a previous trip. Remember, this was the late 60s. These were custom-made Jesus sandals, fitted to footprints drawn on a yellow legal pad in a tiny shop up the stairs in an alleyway midway the block. Winston and I picked up our sandals, put them on, dropped our shoes off at the car, and met up with the friends at a bar. I had never been to a bar before. I was along for the ride and wanted desperately to fit in. Before I knew it, I was introduced to Miller High-Life. I didn't like the taste. I did like how animated I became. I was fitting it. I was funny and part of the group. It was all good- until the ride back to Greensboro. Somewhere between Chapel Hill and Elon College, it happened. I got sick as a dog. Fortunately, I was sitting in the back seat of Winston's brother's Buick (on loan for the weekend). Winston stopped the car, and Tad got my head out the door just in time. I left the better part (or the worst part) of my evening in Chapel Hill alongside the road that night.

I remember waking up the following day lying across my bed in Cox Hall, clothes still damp and my sandals nicely conforming to my feet. (We had been instructed to soak our feet in our new sandals and let them dry while still on our feet so they could shape to the form.) I learned that Winston and the guys had put me in the shower down the hall and then put me to bed- wet from head to sandal. I loved those sandals, and I wore them for years. I never reprised the remainder of that trip. I never developed a taste for the brew and never repeated that choice. To this day, I occasionally enjoy a good glass of wine and have been known to nurture a snifter of brandy or cognac late at night when sitting alone after Becky has called it a day. Some of my best reflections occur during these times.

As the semester wound down, the schoolwork did not get any easier. And, the world, in general, wasn't making any more sense. The semester was ending, and I was perplexed. I knew I wasn't doing as well in school as I had expected, or as I knew I could do. Abroad the war in Vietnam was raging. Domestically, the racial tensions were not getting any better. The presidential election year was getting into full swing. Then, on the evening of April 4th, it exploded. Martin Luther King was assassinated on the balcony of his hotel in Memphis, TN. He had been there leading a protest in support of the sanitation workers. James Earl Ray shot him when he returned to his hotel that evening. It didn't take long for the streets across the country to be filled with angry, primarily young, Black men and women. It was 1968, and the presence of white protesting supporters had not yet risen to the levels we are apt to see these days. (Their presence seemed to be reserved for the anti-war protests). Go back and look at some of the tv coverage of the events. We only had the basic three networks (ABC, CBS, and NBC) back then. Even then, with that limited number of outlets, you got nearly around-the-clock coverage of events. I remember Bud and I deciding we needed to "get out of town." I don't know how to say this. Although I (and I believe Bud as well) was sympathetic to the message of MLK and the plight of our Black brothers and sisters, I was never a marcher. I didn't march against the war. I don't know whether I was (have always been) afraid to step out at those times. I don't know if I didn't "believe in the cause," or was just scared. At any rate, Bud and I decided the next day to leave Greensboro. It was a weekend. Exams would be coming up in just a couple or three weeks. Things were getting dicey in Greensboro. There were rumors students from NC A&T were going to march through Greensboro all the way to Guilford. We didn't want to be there if that happened. Another student, Peter Allen, from Boone, was going home for the weekend. He agreed to give us a ride there. Bud's cousin, Bailey Lowe, was in school at Appalachian State in Boone. Bud called her dorm and asked if we could visit. She said yes, and off we went. It didn't occur to us that we didn't have a ride to Greensboro as Peter was coming back at a different time from when we wanted to return. We would deal with that later.

Off we went. Peter dropped us at the dorm and Bailey met us there. She had arranged for us to stay in one of the men's dorms with a friend whose roommate had left for the weekend. I can't remember much about those 24 hours or so in Boone. We arrived a little after lunch. I couldn't tell you what we did the rest of the day. I recall something about an App State base-ball game- not sure. I began to realize something that should have already been all too clear. Bailey did not feel about me the way I felt about her. We had dated during our senior year in high school. We went to the post-football and basketball game sock-hops. I would see her at church on Sundays. I would call her sometimes at night. That was always an awkward experience.

Our little apartment at Fairview had no privacy. I would take the phone, with its landline, as far as down the short hallway as the cord would reach. Then after the call, Mama would glare at me and want to know what was so secret I had to hide around the corner down the hall. I hated that, but I craved hearing Bailey's voice. If my emotions had not blinded me, I should have seen she was not in the same place I was.

The afternoon and evening and the morning the next day came and went. Mid-afternoon the next day, Bud and I realized it was time to return to Guilford. We had decided the night before that we had no choice. We would hitchhike back. One of Bailey's friends took us to the highway at the edge of the campus. What happened next has stuck with me like it was yesterday. We didn't think about the danger of what we were doing. But, again, this was 1968, and Martin Luther King had just been assassinated. The roads then were different from today. Coming out of Boone was a narrow two-lane country road with little in the way of civilization around it. We were standing on the road, waiting for someone to pick us up. There was little traffic in either direction. (App State wasn't quite the campus then it is today). What little traffic we saw was going toward the campus, not away from it.

I don't know how long we walked. I realized it was getting dark at some point, and we were in the middle of nowhere. You can imagine what went through my mind. It was dark. We were walking alongside a lonely country road in the mountains of North Carolina. The much-beloved leader of the march for human rights, specifically equal civil rights for people of color, had been violently killed less than 96 hours earlier. What had we been thinking? Who knew who might come by and suddenly stop? Well, I knew what I had been thinking. I was in love! No- I mean it! I was in love. It was not a passing fancy. It was not just the usual cravings of the flesh of an 18-year-old American college boy. It was a love that would never be returned and consummated. (After that weekend, I would only see Bailey sparingly over the years, generally, when we would be in Goldsboro on the same weekend.)

Finally, well after the fullness of darkness had descended upon us, a car blew by us and came to a screeching halt. I was at once thrilled to think we were finally going to get back to school. Then just as suddenly, as the car backed towards us and we walked forward, it crossed my mind- oh my God, are they going to kill us? But there we were. There was nowhere to run, and we needed a ride. The yellow Plymouth Duster stopped its backward crawl. The front passenger's seat window came down. "Where y'all going?" Bud, by far the more adventurous of us, replied, "Greensboro, Guilford College- or at least as far in that direction as you can take us."

"Git on in. I'm headed to Raleigh." We got in, and off he went. The driver was youngish, maybe early thirties. He looked a little scruffy, with a few days-old beard and a cigarette hanging from the corner of his mouth. It turns out he didn't have much to say. Bud and I settled down in a few minutes, believing we would not be killed and left in a ditch in the North Carolina mountains. We were able to get to that place because another, equally frightening, possibility quickly emerged. This guy was going to get us all killed. I don't know whether he had been drinking or not. I'm sure he wasn't drunk. I'm not sure he wasn't a little high! We quickly experienced his heavy foot. I don't know the expected driving time between the outskirts of Boone, NC, and the Guilford College exit in Greensboro in the spring of 1968. From the moment Bud and I planted our butts in those black seats in the yellow Duster, that son-of-a-gun headed to Raleigh like a bat out of Hell. The conversation was sparse. I remember speeding through the curves of the highway of downtown Winston-Salem (there was no bypass in those days) at 75 miles mph.

We were nearing the Guilford College exit on Interstate 40 in just a few minutes. We reminded the fellow this was our stop. He screeched to a halt again, and out we jumped. We thanked him for the ride, and without a word, off he sped. I've often wondered whatever happened to that kind soul. In the Bible, Jesus talked about doing unto and for the least of these. That night, in the dark hills of Appalachia, that unknown stranger, in his quiet and seemingly reckless way, certainly did it for two of the least of these. I can't remember his name. I'll never forget his kindness.

Bud and I were back on campus and the semester ended. I finished it and headed home to a summer of work and pining. I never saw Bailey again romantically, and only sporadically later in life. Her memory takes root during this time. Down the road, some three years later, I would meet the woman I fell in love with, and, at the time of this writing, she has been my bride for 51 years and the mother of two wonderful grown children. I have told her much of my growing up years, including high school and Bailey Lowe. Becky, my wife, is an amazing woman in many ways, and you will hear about some of them later. For now, I am reminded of how lovingly she reacted to my sharing some of that time in my life; and being honest with her about how deeply I felt for Bailey and how much it hurt to know the relationship would never evolve and mature. After apologizing to Becky on some occasion, many years ago, when I mentioned Bailey, she stopped me cold in my tracks. "Don't apologize," she told me. "The man I love is at least the sum of all his life experiences and relationships. I like to think you are who you are in no small way due to the love and nurture you expressed in that time. The hurt you felt and learned to absorb has helped mold you into the man I chose to share my life with. I have not been disappointed." I've never been disappointed by Becky. But, much of my life has revolved around one disappointment after another. It sort of became a theme.

I had two jobs that summer. I worked at Wilber's on weekends and occasional weekday catering events. Bud helped me get a weekday job at a moving supply company. We sliced into assorted sizes of damaged newspaper rolls (the rolls newspaper printers put on big printing machines and produce the daily newspaper). We packaged the resulting paper to be used by movers as package stuffing, along with various size cardboard boxes, tape, and other packaging supplies. We shipped them out by tractor-trailer to moving companies from Virginia to South Carolina. There was nothing exotic about it. It was a job for the summer, though, and it paid well. It sure beat cropping tobacco. Working conditions were good, and the people we worked with were pleasant. The company owner and his family were all active members in the Quaker meeting in Goldsboro. Bud had known them all his life and had worked there before. I met them all the year before when I started attending the Meeting after my return from Barbourville.

Shortly after we got home and started working, the country experienced another shock. Remember, this was a presidential election year. The country was in the throes of the anti-Vietnam War movement and the civil rights protests (and sometimes riots). It looked like Robert Kennedy, the younger brother of JFK who had been assassinated barely 1000 days into his presidency, was on track to win the Democratic nomination. That would not be the case. After making a campaign appearance, Robert Kennedy was assassinated in a Los Angeles hotel. His assassin, Sirhan Sirhan, was captured alive on the scene. Much of the conversation Bud and I would engage in the rest of the summer at work touched on various aspects of all these big problems. We occasionally ventured off to what we wanted to do after college. I don't know whether either of us imagined neither would return to Guilford College after the upcoming year.

Sometime during that summer, I bought my first car. I didn't have any money-only what I was making in these summer jobs. I desperately wanted a car. Bud helped me find one. One of Bud's sisters had a car for sale- a Nash Rambler. I paid $500 for it, maybe $400. I'm not sure. All I know is I had a car- at least for a while. That sucker lasted me through the summer and one and a half trips back to Guilford. I drove it back to school and home at Christmas when summer was over. When I left to return to Greensboro after Christmas, I made it as far as the east side of Guilford County. It was dead; the engine was blown. I had been feeding it oil as much as I could. It just drank oil faster than gasoline. Somehow, I managed to get to the college with my duffle bag and suitcase. I had a towing company get it and haul it to a local gas station. In a few days, when I learned what it would cost to fix it, I just had to junk it. My brother and brother-in-law drove up from Goldsboro to take care of everything. I was angry that Bud's sister had sold me a lemon. I was disappointed that I was off to college again and had no car.

My brother and I were never close. He was nearly eighteen years older than me. He was the oldest of five, with me the youngest. Our three sisters were in between. My first memory of

Buddy was when he returned from the Korean War. I must have been four or five years old. After the incident with the Nash Rambler, Buddy came through for me. I didn't say anything to him about it, but I'm sure he could tell how disappointed I was. While I was home for fall break the following October, he arranged for us, with Mama coming along, to look at some used cars. A cousin owned a used car lot between Goldsboro and Wilson. We found a 1964 Chevrolet Chevelle I liked a lot. Buddy did the haggling and got us a reasonable price. Mama had arranged with another cousin to meet with a banker friend to secure a loan with payments I swore I could manage with part-time work back in Greensboro. That cousin, Arnold Jones, co-signed the loan. I would never have gotten the loan without his signature. Buddy and Mama, and I drove back to the lot that same week, and I drove back to Guilford with my 'new" car.

I was back at school, and what was to be a crazy year of highs and lows and next steps and failures was quickly underway. Once again, I was a manager and trainer for the football team. When I arrived at Guilford a year earlier, that was what drove me to want to be there. I knew that was my route to a proper education to prepare me for graduate work in physical therapy and a career in sports medicine- I would be a professional athletic trainer at some big university or even a professional football team. This time back on campus, none of that "rush" was there. I knew none of that was going to happen. It was little more than a work-study job to help make my car payment. School was paid for between need-based scholarships (the merit ones were for one year only) and federal student loans. I needed the job to make the car payment and have a social life. A social life required cash on hand.

So, the semester was underway, and I was going through the motions regarding football. I was more interested in deciding why I was there at all if pursuing a trainer career was no longer the goal. I needed to declare a major, so I did- sociology. I wasn't sure what that was. I knew enough about it to think I could do OK. I could BS with the best of them, at least on paper (my introversion did not allow me to be too spontaneous and vocal in classroom debate situations.) I have no idea how I managed to carry my end of the bargain in Heather Del Aqua's class the previous year. Somehow, that was different. There I was, a sociology major, and beginning to have thoughts about becoming a Quaker minister. When I look back on that year, I wonder, what in the world was I thinking? At any rate, there I was. In a short period, I started down the path of one bad choice after another, with nobody to blame but myself. I didn't break any laws or fall back to alcohol after that drive back from Chapel Hill. No, I just found myself withdrawing from the world I sensed myself failing in, putting on a disguise, and appearing to manage well in that other world. I began cutting classes. I wasn't doing the necessary reading and opting out of class assignments. To avoid being embarrassed, I didn't go to classes. Instead of attending class, I would sleep in or watch TV in the dorm lounge. They say we learn from experience. That may be true- but not always a good thing.

The previous spring semester, I learned I could skip class, show up to take scheduled exams and still pass. I took an English literature course under Professor Andre Youngblood. Andrew was a nice enough man, but an incredibly dull lit professor. He would only read in class excerpts from assigned readings. After a few weeks of the semester, I began cutting classes. Over the semester, I discovered that if I read the material and believed in my BS ability, I could show up and take exams and do well. My final grade in the class was better than my mid-term. That was a terrible lesson to learn. When I returned for the fall 1968 semester and started running into issues, I fell back into that default behavior. The problem was that I didn't have professors in the psychology, sociology, religion, and political science classes I took who were like Andre Youngblood. Eventually, I was cutting classes and no longer trying to keep up with the reading or showing up for exams. I'm not stupid, but you couldn't tell that from my behavior. (Now, even as I sit here writing this and thinking about how ridiculous that behavior was, I do so, acting as if I learned from it and never behaved that way again. Oh- how I wish that were so.)

While disappearing from classes and trying to avoid students I would typically see in those classes, I continued in other venues as if nothing was happening. I forgot to mention this earlier. At the end of the previous spring semester, I had been elected Vice-president of our class. Go figure! Remember, a couple of chapters back, I wrote about high school and being selected as Senior Superlative- Best Personality. Here it was again. I was very likable. I was not the life of the party. I was friendly to everyone- at a distance. I worked at not offending anybody. I wanted to be liked, and I was. So, I performed my duties as class VP. I got a part-time job at the private air terminal at the regional airport near the campus. I worked late afternoons and early evenings a couple of days each week and occasionally Saturday mornings. I've wished many times I had applied myself more to that opportunity. But, having managed to get the job, I wasn't about to ask for anything else. I just showed up and did what I was assigned to do.

I had learned that lesson well from my days in The Project, especially the early days before my Daddy left. I got a second job as the Youth Director at Winston-Salem Friends Meeting (WSFM). The former pastor in Goldsboro, Willie Frye, was now the pastor in Winston-Salem. I would attend the meeting on Sunday mornings and conduct the youth group's activities on Sunday evenings and other occasional outings. I loved Wille and his family and the opportunity he gave me. He knew I was toying with pursuing full-time Quaker ministry, and this experience would benefit me. And, for the most part, it was. I just couldn't help screwing it up.

It was a good size youth group with both junior and senior high school kids and an even mixture of boys and girls. I got along well with all of them. The mother of one of them would later be of significant help when I needed to secure employment to fulfill my Conscientious Objector obligation. The problem was that one of the high school girls was way too assertive regarding things she wanted. She came from a family of substantial means. She was a stellar student. And she was gorgeous. With a mid-October birthday, I was always one of the youngest kids in my classes at school. So here, in the fall of my second year of college, I just turned nineteen. I was barely two years older than the seniors in this group. Let me say right up front, we never "crossed any lines." We spent a lot of weekend time together. I would call her during the week from a payphone at the airport. In those days, long before cell phones, it was a long-distance call. The airport had payphones that were local for either Greensboro, High Point, or Winston-Salem.

For the younger readers, I know that all seems foreign. It was not a good or proper relationship for a Youth Director to have with a student in his youth group. I was a shy nineteen-year-old college guy, and this beautiful, wealthy, smart high school senior was playing the game. I was stupid enough to join in. I can only imagine what might have transpired had she been willing; or had I been more convincing. So, it all didn't end well when her parents forbade her to see me anymore. I didn't think so then, but they were smart enough to know the whole thing was not a good idea.

That was a difficult time for Wille and WSFM. It was the fall of 1968 and the spring of 1969. The Vietnam War raged, and the racial unrest in the country was still raw. By the end of the year, I had begun to question whether Quaker pastoral ministry was a legitimate option for me. I watched firsthand as a long-standing Quaker Meeting tore itself asunder over these issues. I remember a cold winter day when there was a national march against the war. Participants in Winston-Salem planned their route, taking them right by the meetinghouse. We had a handful of folks from the meeting participating. The rub came when the meeting was asked to provide coffee, doughnuts, and a rest stop along the route. The debate was as uncivil as any I had ever witnessed. I don't have room to go into it. Nevertheless, the wounds opened, and the battle lines drawn during that debate would remain fresh when the next issue came to a head.

The next issue involved a daycare program using meeting-house space and some equipment during the weekdays. This was an inner-city population for the most- read that- mostly economically disadvantaged Black children. These preschool kids and teachers descended on the property during the week for a safe and affordable daycare experience. On Friday after-noons, they would return everything to its proper place for Sunday's Sunday school classes and nursery—no harm- No foul. There was a cadre of some of the older leadership in the meeting who had opposed the program from its start. They didn't like the notion of this bunch of preschoolers "running around all over the place, making a mess, spilling food, tearing things up, etc." Some might argue these were not the real reasons for the opposition.

Nevertheless, something happened, and I can't recall just what. It came to a boil about the same time as the tensions associated with the anti-war protests. Before I knew what was happening, the meeting was marching at full speed toward dissolution. I watched Willie try to manage the process. I saw what it did to him and his family. There was ultimately a splitting of the meeting. Willie ended up leaving the ministry for a period. Fortunately, as the years passed, he again joined the ranks of Quaker pastors and continued to stand up for the values he believed were central to his Quaker faith. Unfortunately, our paths diverged down different roads as I left Guilford, and he pursued business opportunities. We would reconnect some years later. For that, I am grateful. I regret missing the years in between. Can't get 'em back!

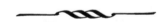

At the time of this writing, I am a man living every day firmly in the throes of old age. It's a fascinating thing. I wake up every day and greet that fact. My hair is gray (I still have an ample supply). My joints ache from time to time. I look at my hands and see a maze of lines and wrinkles. I stand at a urinal and wonder if I will have to pay rent to be there as I have to wait for it all to run its course. Finally, it does. I am not the seventeen-year-old kid

who showed up on campus in the Quacker Box parking lot fifty-five years ago.

Looking back over those two years, I don't know where to begin. How did I get from The Project, an accomplished student with a wide-open future ahead of me, to flunking a class right out of the box and hiding in the dorm TV room? In two short years, how did my hopes and dreams about success, status, and financial stability shatter into a thousand incoherent pieces of a broken future? How did I go from "being in love" to lamenting that I had been unable to see the obvious? How could I abuse the opportunities before me at seventeen and allow them to move on without me?

Could the answer to that question be so simple? I wanted to believe every day revolved around me and my wants. By the time I reached Guilford, I had plenty of evidence this was not the case. Rarely had anything in my life ever revolved around me. How could I be so stupid as to make choices that only sped up the pace of that fracture? Simple! I had seventeen years of hanging onto every thread of hope that, this time, this opportunity, it would finally be my turn. Despite the occasional peaks that justified this optimism, the almost daily visits to the valleys easily clouded out much of the life of optimism. When failure in the biology lab knocked on my door, I was well perched to answer the call. Again, simple!

Just "don't ask for a damn thing," and never let them see you cry. And that's just what I did. I wasn't the first college freshman to mindlessly start down this path. Often, alcohol or some other behavior influencing drugs provide the vehicle to ramp up the pace of the crash. That was not my story. I didn't need a foreign substance to grease the skids. All I needed was the occasionally surfacing, always deeply entrenched, reminder of who I was and what my role was not- "I can't see through muddy water," and repeat, "Don't ask for a damn thing." My role was not to seek advice, help, or guidance (counseling). My role was to avoid taking a position in front. (I don't know how the cheerleader thing ever came about- so out of character).

The paradox here is mind-boggling. After arriving full of hopes, dreams, and aspirations, I found the road much rockier and more uninviting than I imagined. I still managed to present publicly that "Best Personality" pose. The impact of the combined occasional peaks and routinely traversed valleys was quickly hidden. All one has to do is smile at folks, laugh a little, not draw attention, and never argue or be combative. Always give in.

Now, fifty-four years later, I must acknowledge that the two-year slide downhill produced far more peaks than valleys; that is, consequences directly related to that window of time. However, what keeps me returning to the question at hand is how to deal with all the other valleys after that brief period. What does one do when he knows intellectually right from wrong, good choices from bad choices, and yet, makes the wrong choices anyway? What in one's psyche allows (causes?) him to behave in a way he knows is not in his best interest, yet he does so anyway? During these two years, I wish I had been more responsive to that Inner

Light (as my Quaker friends would describe it). At some point along this road, I wish I had been able to internalize and act accordingly upon the insanity of fearing to ask for help. I wish I had been more willing to accept notice and acclaim for successes and then put in the work to build upon those successes.

Here I sit, a 73-year-old husband, father, grandfather, brother, uncle. Those opportunities have pretty much passed on now. Life is like that. It doesn't wait for you to get on board. The globe turns. The days begin. The days end. Whatever happens in that cosmically brief interval each day is done. Some things get rectified after the fact. For the most part though, tomorrow is a new day. As a younger man, with proper counseling, coaching, and motivation, I might have (in a sense) unheard my Daddy's warnings. But, no- I still hear them today. They ain't going nowhere. I referred to my ongoing faith walk in my letter prefacing this epistle. I wish I had been more decisive in my efforts in that walk in my earlier years when there was time and there were opportunities to demonstrate my ability to put behind me what I learned as a child. Now, at this late date, it just feels like the clock is running out. I'm tired of that struggle. But, the notion of that Inner Light I learned about as a Convinced Friend still lingers. I want to believe that Inner Light still flickers within me!

Chapter 9

DROPPING OUT

BY THE TIME the spring of my second year at Guilford was underway, it was clear I would not be back. I don't remember knowing that at the outset; my behavior demonstrated it. I rarely went to class. I slept in, watched TV, and hid from most social contact. I got a part-time job working at the private air terminal at the regional airport. I continued my work at Winston-Salem Friends Meeting. Although I was on academic probation warning, I was allowed to continue my place on the cheerleading squad. That was the one bright spot of the campus life.

Somewhere about midterm, I drifted into a very dark and dangerous place. That was the only time I consciously thought about suicide as more than a sociological phenomenon. I studied it in class and found the concept understandable. I don't recall having thought about it in a personal sense. Yet, there I was, and it was cropping up in my quiet moments. Looking back on that time, I realize how naïve and silly I was. I remember leaving my dorm room one night and walking over to the baseball field. It was a beautiful starry early spring evening. The baseball field had a grassy knoll along the left field line.

I found myself lying there, holding a whole bottle of aspirin. For the life of me now, I have no idea what prompted that walk with that bottle of aspirin that evening. I don't even know what a bottle of aspirin would do. I thought it was enough to be fatal, painless, and not messy. While I can't remember what triggered that walk, I do remember sitting and lying on that knoll for hours, crying my eyes out. I was alone. I remember thinking no one would miss me. No one would care after a few days. Many would be surprised- folks who had no idea how badly I was failing, failing not just in class but in every aspect of life. By this time, I realized I would not return to Guilford in the fall. If I didn't decide to drop out, the college would do it for me. My mind would take me back to high school, just two short years earlier, and how the future looked so bright and exciting. What would the coaches think? What about those kids I envied so much from high school, kids I wished I could be like and have what they had. I thought about how it would break my mother's heart- a woman who had known so much pain and disappointment.

After several hours on that knoll, I returned to my dorm room. I couldn't do it. I just couldn't do it. Was I too afraid? Or was I too strong? That is a debate I've had with myself many times over the years. I don't know. That would not be the last time those feelings and that debate would rage within me. I'm seventy-three years old now. That evening on the knoll was fifty-four years ago. I can still feel it today. I have often referred to myself as a "sociologist by academic training." That moniker allows me to get away with telling folks I can understand, purely from an academic standpoint, why and how someone can get to that place where ending their life makes sense. I have said that occasionally over the years. It used to worry Becky.

I always assured her it was nothing more than an academic understanding. I could never "go there." If for no other reason, my faith walk and my love for her and my family would not allow me to go there. Finding myself at this keyboard, writing these words, suggests that I was either mistaken or dishonest with myself, or my faith walk has devolved to a point where I no longer view the concept solely through an academic lens. I don't think so. But it does sometimes scare me.

Not long after that night on the knoll, just weeks before spring break, I was aroused from another morning of sleeping in. No one else was in the suite in Bryan Hall, and I could have just stayed in bed. But whoever was knocking would not stop. So, I crawled out and opened the front door. Suddenly, I froze. There stood Pete, a religion professor whose class I had been cutting regularly. I first met Pete when I was assigned to his faculty small group book study. He and I would become friends, particularly after I returned to Guilford as the Director of Financial Aid.

I invited him in. We walked through the common room back to my room. It was a small room with no seating except two desk chairs and two beds. We both sat down on the edge of my unmade bed. Right out of the chute, Pete asked if I was all right. He was concerned I had been missing his class. He had asked some other students about me. They hadn't seen me or heard anything from me. I told him I was OK. I can't recall the contents of much of that conversation. I remember him telling me it is sometimes OK to take a time-out. He said he knew I was capable of a much better profile than the one I was casting. He did not blame me in any way or come across as judgmental. He understood I was struggling with issues far more critical at that moment than any scholarly Old Testament review. Pete was referred to as a "weighty Friend," meaning a Quaker highly regarded and respected in Quaker circles. His footprint was much bigger than just that of a small college religion professor. His words to me were moving. I was then, and still am today, quite taken by the fact that this "weighty Friend" who I admired would care enough to come get me out of bed to ask if I was all right; and talk about options.

During that conversation on the edge of my bed, I began to think about flunking out of Guilford as more than just another failing disappointment in my life. I began to think about plotting a course for what lay ahead after that semester at Guilford. Things began to move quickly. My attention shifted from focusing on failing at college and the disappointment associated with that to figuring out what I would do next and where I would do it. To this day, I am forever grateful for Pete. I don't know how life might have been different had it not been for that saint showing up at my door. He and I would have more conversations about that moment years later when I joined Guilford's staff. He lived in the community and remained a Guilford fixture for many years.

The first order of business was to finish the semester. I could say I returned to my classes and improved my academic performance for the remainder of the semester. That would be a lie. I didn't. It was too late to fix any of that. I finished the semester living in Bryan Hall and eating my meals in the college caf. After all, room and board had been paid for through the end of the semester. During that time, though, I decided to apply for Conscientious Objector status with the Selective Service. The war in Vietnam was still raging. This was one of the things that weighed heavily on me during this period. I was willing to give two years of service, just not in support of that war effort. A whole host of factors drove that decision. The match that lit the fire was seeing a photo of one of my high school friends sent from Vietnam. Ralph Denning was the nicest guy you would ever want to meet. He was funny. He was kind and gentle. Unfortunately, he was also drafted and sent to 'Nam. In this photo, Ralph was standing in a semi-circle with his fellow soldiers in full battle fatigues. Around his neck, Ralph was wearing a necklace made of human ears. I couldn't believe what I saw. The Ralph I had known for years was not the man in that picture. Aside from all the geopolitical issues regarding the war, I decided I could not willingly allow myself to participate in something so vile it could bring out that kind of "worst" in me. I could not let that happen. I decided to apply for CO status and prayed it would be granted. I don't know what I would have done had it not been.

That process itself was stressful. The process involved completing a form, providing two references, and writing a letter, citing the reason(s) for requesting CO status. The Selective Service prescribed a set of circumstances that might qualify one for CO status. One of those circumstances was religious affiliation. The Society of Friends has a long-standing "peace testimony." For that reason, Quakers usually could get through this process with little difficulty. Once status was approved, the CO had to secure a job for two years doing work of a "service" nature that complied with the SS requirements for meeting a national need. Most often, these jobs were in hospitals, schools, libraries, or construction work building these facilities.

In any case, even though I was now a "convinced Friend," had filled the pulpit in the Goldsboro Friends Meeting for three months, and was enrolled at a Quaker college, the local draft board did not see fit to approve my application. I was surprised- and scared to death. When I applied, the decision to leave Guilford was a done deal. I couldn't go back even if I wanted to. So, an appeal of the Wayne County Draft Board's decision was in order. I was allowed to take with me one supporting witness/reference. I took with me Mr. Luby Casey. Mr. Casey (I could never call him Luby, never mind the Quaker tradition of first names) was another one of those "weighty Friends." He was well into his senior status by then. He was a well-known local businessman, a nurseryman. He was a multi-term Trustee of Guilford College. When the time came, he stood up and gave me a wonderful recommendation supporting my application.

The Board understood my Quaker connections. I think they had doubts about my sincerity, given I was a "convinced Friend," not a birthright Friend, having come to the faith just before my senior year in high school. I would not be the first college kid trying to buck the draft in such a manner. I'll never forget our discussion around a particular scenario they posed. The Board asked me to pretend I was married and at home one evening with my wife and two children. It was late at night. We had all gone to bed. I hear noise coming from the living room. I go downstairs and encounter a masked burglar armed with a pistol. He points the gun at me and tells me to lead the way upstairs. What would I do? Would I meekly obey his command, or would I try to disarm him to protect my family, even if that meant possibly bringing harm or death to myself or the intruder?

I must admit. I was prepared for that question. Due to my Quaker connections, I had received some briefing on what to expect in this appeal hearing. Being prepared and responding truthfully and believably are two different things. I told the

Board I did not know what I would do. I didn't know how they could expect an eighteen-year-old kid from The Project to understand what he would do in that scenario. Then I said what I hoped I would do, based on my faith position then. It went something like this. Since this person with the gun was where he was and doing what he was doing, he did not share my Christian values and perspective. While I did not wish to die at that moment, nor did I wish any harm to come to my family, I believed I and my family, based on our faith walk at that time, were ready to "meet our maker," as the saying goes. I didn't welcome the possibility, but I could accept it. On the other hand, this person was likely not in the same position. I could not believe he was ready to "meet his maker." I could not be responsible for sending him down that path, no matter the cause. Likewise, I could not do so within the context of any manufactured war.

The Board members seemed to understand my rather simplistic response. They followed with an offer I had not expected. I don't know whether I missed this part in my earlier Quaker briefings; or if this was something new. At any rate, they asked if I could see myself serving in the army as a non-combatant. If my objection to the service was my unwillingness to commit violence against anyone, why could I not serve as a medic? Then not only would I not be committing violence in the cause of the war, but I would also be saving lives-all kinds of lives- Believers, non -Believers, and other faiths. It took me a minute. I was unnerved by the question and wrestling with how to reply. What would stand in the way of taking that "out"? Then, I saw the picture of Ralph and his necklace of ears. I gathered myself and thanked them for being willing to expand the view. Then I told them a non-combatant role would not be acceptable.

While my training and assigned role would be to bring healing and comfort, once in-country and in the field, I would have little control over what scenarios might unfold. I was fearful of finding myself in a situation where an officer, in dire circumstances, might order me to do something that ran against my beliefs and my training. I suspected, and today I'm sure they knew those real-life situations occur in wartime. I kept seeing Ralph. Whatever he encountered in his days in combat changed him into a person I would not know. I could not willingly allow myself to be placed in such a situation.

So, they denied my appeal. Then I was terrified. By this time, I had been classified 1-A, eligible for service. But, there remained one last level of appeal- the state board of appeals. So, I immediately filed an appeal and, within days, received approval with a new draft status of 1-O, CO status with "service available for civilian work contributing to the maintenance of the national health, safety, or interest."

During this whole CO application process, I believed it would all work out. Wille Frye and Friends at WS Friends Meeting and Cal McGrath, a Quaker pastor in Greensboro, had been incredibly supportive. So, even while going back and forth with the draft board, I pursued options for securing the required two years of "service." In addition, since I would be out of the dorm by mid-May, I needed something to do and somewhere to go for the summer. I did not want to go back to Goldsboro. By this time, Goldsboro had become the place where I grew up; but it was no longer home. I didn't feel like I had a home. No one in my family could relate to what I was doing. I am sure they were disappointed in my dropping out of college. To this day, I have no idea as to whether they knew I had flunked out of college.

Come to the rescue Bud Andrews. Unknown to me at the time, Bud was also planning to leave Guilford at the end of the semester. But instead, he transferred to Campbell College and joined the National Guard the following semester while still enrolled at Campbell. He would graduate from Campbell and make a second career in the NC National Guard, rising to the rank of a full-bird Colonel. We have often joked over the years about this birthright Friend of several generations making a side career in the army while his "convinced Friend" friend volunteered as a Conscientious Objector and worked as a hospital orderly for two years. But I get ahead of myself.

Bud had a great idea and, as it turned out, had already started the ball rolling. Bud asked me if I would be interested in working at Quaker Lake as a camp counselor for most of the summer. Quaker Lake is a beautiful summer camp setting, year-round church retreat, and meeting facility. Bud and I would join several other college students to serve as counselors for eight weeks of summer camp for elementary to high school kids. Those eight weeks were a great buffer, an appropriate transition from my sense of failure at Guilford to anticipating what lay ahead in my next two years. By the time summer camp began, I had secured a placement for my two years of community service. Having that settled, I could focus on my duties and adventures as a church camp counselor. Fifty-four years later, I still reflect on those weeks with fond memories.

My next stop would be Forsyth Memorial Hospital in Winston-Salem. I would go to work as an orderly (I think nowadays it would be a CNA.) I would work in the John C. Whitaker Care Center, the hospital's physical therapy and rehab wing. I am grateful to the member of the WS Friends Meeting who facilitated that placement. She was the mother of a couple of kids in the youth group with which I worked. She was also a senior staff member in the nursing staff at the hospital. When I went to work there, I was the first Conscientious Objector the hospital had hired. By the time I left, nearly two years later, several COs were working to fulfill their Selective Service obligation.

When I moved into one room in a boarding house in Winston-Salem going into this two-year experiment, I had no way of knowing how that decision and the ensuing two years would define the rest of my life. As I have grown older, I have learned that life is a series of choices- big and small- among other things. We can rarely know the long-term result of these choices, mainly because following every choice that sets us on a particular path is a multitude of other decisions- again, big and small- that tweak and shape the effects of that earlier choice. I don't know how life would have evolved differently had I not quit being the student I know I could have been (as evidenced by my performance a few years later). I have some regrets about my decision-making during that time in my life. I don't know that whatever life may have evolved from a different set of decisions would have resulted in a different outlook or mental state. There is just no way of knowing. One can wish and hope things could have been different. As the saying goes- "be careful what you wish for." I know my wife, children, and grandchildren love me. I am in surprisingly good health- no serious maladies. I am not wealthy. I am comfortable. I cannot afford to do many things I wish Becky and I could do. One big regret I have about that time is that, somehow, Bud and I let our paths diverge. It's understandable. We both were dealing with the unexpected rerouting of our lives and career paths in volatile times. Fortunately, we would reconnect, and though we have never spent much time together, we have continued to value our friendship and appreciate what each has contributed to the other's life.

Next stop- Winston-Salem and Forsyth Hospital!

From college to kids' camp, to pushing bedpans and giving enemas- all in four months. Life is a collection of moments and memories, choices and consequences, people, places, and things. How many of us can honestly surmise that our position in this thing we call life is what and where we envisioned it to be years ago? How many of us understood how much or how little control we have over the moments, the choices, the people, places, and things we encountered along the way? We plan- maybe. We study-maybe. We prepare-maybe. Ultimately, are we not often victims of circumstances well beyond our control? Is how our lives evolve and progress not as much a result of how we react to life as how we plan, study, and prepare to be in charge of our lives? These months saw my life take a sharp turn from college, with all its built-in ambitions and goals, to performing menial labor in a hospital ward, with a sense of failure and lost direction. How much of that sharp turn should have been a surprise to anyone? Was it even a sharp turn? Or was it a logical progression of events resulting from a long history of choices and devalued self-esteem? The new direction embarked upon in the summer of 1969 was at least as predictable as any other expectation about academic success preceding that time.

The point is that many variables always direct, or at least impact, one's life. The months leading up to my separation from Guilford College and pivoting to the next episode in life were not, in themselves, responsible for that transition. No, the timeframe is much longer than that. For purposes of this exercise, let's agree that the moments, the choices, and the people, places, and things that stood front and center during this brief window of time were no more impactful on the saga that is still unfolding than those that occurred or were present years earlier. They all seem to build upon one another. Bottom line– I don't know how much control any of us have over all of this. At best, maybe we play in the margins. Sometimes we "learn our lesson" and perhaps alter future developments in some positive way. This sounds fatalistic. I hate that. That is where I find myself all too often. How to bend that curve?

Chapter 10

AN UNEXPECTED GLIMMER

QUAKER LAKE AND its wealth of memories came to an end. I had to leave before the final week of camp to report to my new job at the hospital. I was in for a radical change in routine and lifestyle. I moved into a boarding house in the West End neighborhood near downtown Winston. There were only three or four boarders with the husband-and-wife owners living downstairs. It was an old house in a neighborhood that, in its day, had been a very upscale part of the near-downtown residential community. The thing I remember most about it was it had an elevator. When you counted the basement and the attic, the house had four floors. My room was on the fourth floor. They had converted the attic into two rooms for rent. We (the boarders) were not allowed to use the elevator though. A few years after my time in the house, the owners sold it to a young lawyer and his family. It became a part of the next phase of neighborhood development. Many of these old houses were sold to younger, more financially affluent folks who launched a significant revitalization of that area- not without some pushback from more traditionalists, I'm sure.

I had just one room. There was a refrigerator outside my door which I shared with another boarder. I was allowed a hot plate, no other cooking appliance. The hospital was only a five-minute drive from my room. The meeting house was a few minutes away and convenient for my continued work there. I could have friends visit, but I had to keep the door open if they were female friends. That was OK. I didn't have friends other than folks from the church, and they were not coming to my room.

The work schedule was a rude awakening for me. Anyone who has ever done shiftwork in a hospital will know what I mean. I am not a morning person. I have never been. I can stay up 'til midnight and beyond. Over the years, I have always had to be up earlier than I would prefer. This was my first encounter with routinely being at work at 6:45 in the morning. And if that wasn't enough of an adjustment, even that wasn't the complete picture. My work schedule would change every six weeks. It would go from working the first shift (7-3) to the second or third shift (3-11 or 11-7).

To make matters worse, it was not a Monday through Friday deal. No- it might be Monday-Thursday with two days off and four or five days on before, three days off. I had been informed that this kind of rotating day schedules and shifts is expected in that arena. So, I was aware of it; but I wasn't prepared for it. Like so many things in life, you learn to adapt and move on. I got into the flow easily enough. Most of the folks I worked with were friendly enough. I had expected some pushback, given my CO status. I did not know at first who knew my circumstances for being there. I learned soon enough that most of the nursing staff knew. They treated me like the other orderlies (or female aides). Other than some of the specific duties the job required to maintain patients' cleanliness, it was not all that bad. Given the nature of the facility (a longer-term physical therapy and rehab caseload), patients would often be in our care for months at a time. During my two years there, I became a friend, not just a caregiver, to several patients.

For the most part, days (or evenings, depending on the shift) became routine. That experience taught me that injury, illness, and disease do not discriminate. I served patients from all walks of life and all socio-economic sectors. It was a job, and I performed it at a high standard. Some patients touched me in ways that have stayed with me over the years. A few come to mind. There was a young Black woman who had rheumatoid arthritis. She must have been in her thirties. I do not know how long she had been in the condition she was when I first met her. She was small in stature and build. Her tiny body was frozen in almost a fetal position. Arthritis had contracted her muscles and bones to such a point. Times are different now, and the growth of specialized facilities outside primary care hospitals has led to patients such as Faye being moved to these facilities for what, often, is the remainder of their lives. In Faye's case, she was at Whitaker for most of my two years there.

While I was not called upon to provide any intimate personal care due to gender considerations, I was often called to assist with linen changes and lift Faye so the aides could do whatever they needed to do. Sometimes, particularly on third shift, she would call me to her room to get her a sip of water. If I wasn't busy with other patients, we would just visit. She was such a sweet person. I do not remember ever seeing her in a down or foul mood. She was a woman of immense faith. I've often wondered how she could be so strong in her Christian faith while being trapped with the physical existence that she was. There are many things in life I do not understand. Now, I don't know what she thought about or cried about every hour of every day. I know I never witnessed any behavior remotely suggestive of anything other than a beautiful young woman of God. I have spent many hours over the years reflecting on Faye and trying to imagine.

Another patient I grew to enjoy spending time with was an older Black man. Robert, like Faye, was a patient for an extended time. Robert had a severe stroke. He was paralyzed but had regained some degree of his speech. I would stop by Robert's room when time allowed, and we would talk. Unlike Faye, Robert never had any visitors. He wasn't quite the "man of God" as Faye was a "woman of God." He was a kind and gentle soul. He just was a little more earthy in nature. I'll never forget one night he couldn't sleep, which was not unusual.

As I walked by his room, he called out loud to me. "Mr. Gurley," he called. I popped into the room and asked what I could do for him. He wanted a cup of coffee. I called the nurse's station to make sure it was OK to give him coffee at that time of the night. It was. So, I asked him how he liked it- black, sugar, sweetener, cream. He got the biggest grin on his face with those pearly white teeth and said, "I like my coffee just like I like my women- black and strong." I cracked up. And he did too. We got the biggest laugh out of that. I told him I had never heard that expression before. He said, "Well, it's true- black and strong." I told him I'd get him a cup. I couldn't vouch for its strength, but it would be black. I would share many such coffee visits with Robert over the ensuing months. I missed him when he was transferred. I visited him a few times after his relocation before he died from a respiratory infection. I can still see that beautiful smiling face.

I would be remiss if I did not share the story of Stan and Larry. Stan and Larry shared a room at the end of the hall on the first floor of the JCWCC. Stan was an eighteen-year-old recent high school graduate from just north of Winston-Salem, and Larry was a sixteen-year-old high school kid from north of Durham. Stan was a paraplegic, and Larry, a quadriplegic. Both were patients at the center for most of my time there. It is important to note the age similarity between me and these guys. After first meeting Stan and Larry, it didn't take long to become friends. In those days, patients would complete a menu selection form with each morning's breakfast for the next day's meals.

I never had any money during those two years. I learned how to be a good shopper and find bargains. Somehow Stan and Larry got wind of my financial plight (we did talk a lot about "stuff.") They started asking me what I wanted for breakfast. Then, one would order extra milk and cereal for the next day. The other would order an extra cinnamon roll or toast. Sometimes there would be an extra juice or piece of sausage or bacon. For months many of my breakfasts came from these guys- maybe a little late in the morning when I could take my morning break- but free. I was indeed grateful. In this vein, I learned where the food bargains were, all-you-can-eat buffets where I could have supper and not need to eat again for a day or two. I knew where you could buy one, get one free, and use the fridge outside my room door at the boarding house to save it. I learned to enjoy pork & beans, beanie-weenies (still do today), peanut butter, and where to buy day-old bread and sweets.

Stan was a three-sport athlete in high school and was weeks away from enrolling at NC State University, planning to be an architect, when he suffered a catastrophic injury on a construction site in his hometown. He fell through an unfinished skylight on a residential construction project. As a result of the accident, Mike was permanently paralyzed from the waist down.

Larry was completely paralyzed from the neck down. He was injured in a car accident coming home from a day at Kerr Lake with his brother and a friend. Larry had been lying in the back seat of his brother's car when they came out of a fog bank only to see a jack-knifed tractor-trailer truck ahead of them. They collided with the trailer. Larry was the only one seriously injured.

The bond the three of us formed during those months is hard to describe. Both young men were Believers and unabashed about expressing their faith. They were also typical small-town American high schoolers. They enjoyed talking about sports and girls- not necessarily in that order. In addition to the routine care and maintenance required in my job description, I would get them up and take them for rides around the campus. This was one of the highlights of their days- getting outside, breathing fresh air. They regularly left the room to go to PT. *We* went outside. We would share meals when my schedule allowed. I would visit them on days off and bring a special snack when I came across a bargain.

Larry's condition was such that his realistic expectations were limited. Remember, this was 1969-71. Much of the computer and mechanical technology available to broaden the horizons of individuals in Larry's situation did not exist then. Larry had a wonderful attitude, and we worked hard to encourage progress.

Stan, permanently paralyzed from the waist, had different horizons ahead of him. He was going to PT. After a few months of therapy, he was not making the kind of progress his doctors and therapists expected. Nothing about his physical condition precluded his making better strides toward moving out of the treatment facility and even resuming his college ambitions. Progress was not happening. I reported to work one Monday after being off for three days. It didn't take long to realize something was different about Stan. After Stan had returned from his daily PT session and my shift for the day ended, I stopped in to tell him and Larry to have a good evening and that I would see them for breakfast in the morning. Before I left, I had to ask Stan what had happened over the weekend. I told him I sensed something different. I'll never forget the smile that came over his face.

Stan got a little teary-eyed and paused for a minute. Then he shared. His youth pastor from back home had come to visit on Saturday. That was not unusual. He was a regular visitor every couple of weeks. During this visit, the matter of Stan's PT progress, or lack thereof, came up. The pastor said something to Stan I have never forgotten. I have used this story on numerous occasions to get to a point. The way Stan told it, in response to asking his youth pastor, "What else can I do?" the youth pastor told him this, and I quote, "Stan, you're a young man that can't walk. You are, nonetheless, a Man."

When Stan repeated those words, I could see the pastor had spoken to the depths of Stan's soul. It was never about Stan's ability to do the physical work required to re-enter life outside the facility. It was about the "why" he should put forth that effort since he believed his existence as a man had been forever truncated. He was never going to live life as he, the three-sport star, had envisioned it. Life, as he dreamed it, was gone. The youth pastor's words hit him hard, in a positive way. He was not dead. His future was not gone. Life, love, and the pursuit of happiness (my words, not his) were still there for him to experience. His path now would have to differ from what he perceived a few months earlier. There was a good path that could bring the same kinds of love, life, and happiness he thought had been taken away from him.

From that day forward, the pace of his physical development escalated. He had a new understanding of his future and was willing to invest the physical, mental, and emotional capital to make it happen.

I must back up a bit and add a wrinkle to the story. As I said, Stan, Larry, and I became more than patients and caregiver. We became friends and even confidants. Remember I said we enjoyed talking about girls and sports (yes, in that order.) One of the things I enjoyed about working at the hospital was the school of nursing affiliated with it. Most of that education has been transferred to colleges and community colleges for years. Back then, many large community hospitals had their own school of nursing. In addition to their classroom and laboratory training, students would spend a required number of hours each term gaining clinical experience in various hospital areas. By the time they graduated, they would have worked on the floors everywhere in the hospital, from emergency to surgery, from labor & delivery to physical therapy and rehab-getting firsthand exposure and experience with actual patients and nursing staffs and organizational behavior. At Whitaker, we would see students from the hospital's nursing school and from across town at the Wake Forest University-owned Baptist Hospital School of Nursing. I looked forward to the days these students would be on the floor.

It was bound to happen sooner or later. I have always been shy and introverted about making conversation and taking the first step. One afternoon I was sitting at the nurse's station. My work was caught up, and I was waiting for the next call from a room needing something. Suddenly, walking down the hall toward Stan and Larry's room was the cutest thing I had ever seen. She was one of the student nurses. We had met briefly previously. When on their clinical rotations, students would be assigned to designated patients. This angel walking down the hall had been assigned to Stan and Larry. I don't remember when, but at some point, I had been called in to assist this student with getting Larry onto a bedpan. It was all very professional and a routine part of the job. But I was struck!

The next day after seeing her going to the guys' room on her day off, wearing a leopard pattern jumpsuit (and wearing it very well), I mentioned it to the guys. I told them she was the most beautiful thing I had ever seen. I told them I would love to get to know her. I was so shy though; it would never happen. Well- that set the table for the two of them. Little did I know then, they took it upon themselves to take on the role of Cupid. Whenever she worked in their room, they would go out of their way to mention "Mr. Gurley." They would build me up and suggest I might be interested in asking her out. When I was with the guys, they would encourage me to get up the nerve. All the while, life, and work went on. I would see her going up and down the halls and would occasionally actually encounter her on the job in a professional capacity. I don't remember the timeframe. I do remember trying to offer her a ride on her walk to a park near the students' residence hall. I didn't usually go by it on my drive to and from work; until, by accident, I discovered she enjoyed going there to read. Suddenly, I found a new regular route to and from work. She never did allow me to pick her up though. This all transpired during the winter of 1970-71.

For the life of me, I cannot recall how I managed to get her phone number. Remember, this was long before cell phones and social media. I remember calling the nursing students' residence hall, trying to reach her. She wasn't there. She had gone home for the weekend, which was normal behavior for her. Whoever I spoke with, maybe her roommate, gave me her number.

This part I do remember well. It was late morning or early afternoon on Saturday, February 28th, 1971. Frozen, and almost speechless, I called her at home. Here I was, calling this creature that had stolen my heart, and we had never even been alone together. When she came to the phone, I managed to stumble through a couple of sentences of small talk and then asked the question. Guilford College had a good men's basketball program, and they were playing Winston-Salem State University that evening in the Winston-Salem Coliseum. I didn't know whether she had a regular boyfriend or not. I didn't know whether she liked sports or not. (I would learn, not too much later, she had been well immersed in a sports culture all her life, particularly baseball.) I asked her for a first date just hours before the game started. Somehow, I managed to get the words out, and to my amazement, she said, "Yes." Sitting here writing this, some fifty-four years later, I can feel my heart pound, just the sheer joy of the memory of that moment. Little could I imagine what that "yes" would translate into over the next weeks and months...and years. I had no way of knowing she did have a regular boyfriend. Earlier that day, he had called and canceled a date for that evening- and that did not sit well with her. So, she said "yes" to me to 'get even' with him. I knew none of this at the time. Sometime later, when that story came out, I wanted to find this guy and thank him. I never did.

I hung up the phone and could hardly breathe. It's interesting how some things from that period are little more than vague blurs in my memory. Others are as vivid and visceral as if they were happening all over again. I welcome that feeling. I've missed it too much in my life.

From that point, I only remember getting my car washed before returning to my room. By this time, I had moved from the boarding house on Summit Street to a room in a small house closer to downtown. It was just me and the landlady, an elderly widow who rented the room mainly to have some company in the house at night. It gave her a sense of security.

After returning to my room, I waited impatiently for the afternoon to pass. Finally, it was time to clean up, dress, and drive to Kernersville. Over the years, I had passed the signs at the off-ramps to Kernersville hundreds of times between Greensboro and Winston-Salem. I had never been to Kernersville- a small town with barely a stoplight back then. I didn't get to Kernersville proper that evening. It turned out she lived on a farm. That evening introduced me to the family that would become my second home and the town that would become my permanent address for decades to come. And, in many ways, I gained a father I never had.

I had no idea what to expect. I didn't know Becky came from a farm family, and I was heading to the country. She had given me directions over the phone- remember, again, no map quest or Google Maps back then. I found her house, parked, and went to the door to call for her. I remember spending little time with introductions beyond the basics. I do remember finding myself almost breathless when she came into the room. She wore a beige sweater-type dress with a multiple-colored striped shirt. She wore brown shoes with big buckles across the bridge. I'm not kidding- I could hardly catch my breath. I know folks use the expression "love at first sight" somewhat whimsically.

I am here to tell you that is what I was experiencing. (Tears are welling up even now as that image floats through my mind while editing this text.) I first felt it weeks earlier when I saw her walking down the hall in the Whitaker Care Center. I would be less than candid if I pretended some of what I was feeling was not what any twenty-year-old all-American male would have felt, seeing what I was seeing. Yes- that is true. At that moment, I knew what I was feeling was way more than that. Now, fifty-two years later, I still get that feeling. I still have to catch my breath sometimes. It hasn't all been fun and roses; It has been a deep, abiding love I could only imagine that afternoon on the steps of her back porch. AUTHOR'S NOTE: It was not "love at first sight" for Becky. It took her a bit longer. She still had this boyfriend to deal with. Stan and Larry had work to do. Somehow though, it all came together. Slightly over four months from that first date on February 28th, on July 4th, I would ask her to marry me. She said "yes" again. I was on a roll.

When Becky said "yes," I knew I had to finish my CO obligation and return to school. I petitioned the draft board to allow me to leave CO placement a few weeks early to re-enter Guilford in August. They approved, and Guilford re-admitted me. Becky had one more year in nursing school. So, I set about returning to school that fall. Becky continued her nursing program, and together we began planning for a wedding the following summer, after her graduation. We were married on June 18th, 1972, Father's Day. What a cruel joke to play on Royce Smith, my new father-in-law. I could not have married into a family that could have welcomed me as a son any more than Royce and Peggy Smith. Whatever demons, disappointments, and failures I have struggled with in my adult years have in no way been attributable to either my wife or these beautiful people.

Leaving Guilford two years earlier after experiencing failure in a way I had never known was a painful and embarrassing time. I launched into the two years obligation assuming it would be a total waste of time. Without that diversion on my life's path, I would never have seen that beautiful creature in the leopard jumpsuit walking down the hall. There is nothing in this world I would take for that moment and all the moments with her since then. Therein lies the dilemma. I know in my heart I have been blessed immeasurably by the love of my life and the children that came out of that blessing. Of that, I am certain. Still, when my mind moves to that place where I begin weighing successes and failures, material losses and gains and comparisons, performance success and shortcomings- it is hard to focus on the blessings. Are those deeply rooted blessings, which don't always take front and center in the moment, strong enough to outweigh the recurring, seemingly, ever-present sense of failure and disappointment? Often, the answer to that question is a shattering "No!" So, the dilemma nags and gnaws.

For this moment, though, life was good, and Becky provided more than an unexpected glimmer of hope.

This entire process has been a lot of things; informative, taxing, thought-provoking, and evocative. This brief two-year period stimulates several observations and raises even more questions. Until my leaving home to go to college, with the exception (and a big exception it was) when my father walked out and the timing of that departure, my life had been stable. There had been few changes in routine,

surroundings, culture, and social connections. I grew up in a town of less than 30,000 people. From first grade through high school, I went to school with almost all the same people. There was some infusion of new faces from the Air Force base when we got to high school. My first year attending school with students of color was my junior year in 1965. My days living in that small eastern North Carolina town changed little from when I was old enough to participate in any socialization process to when my mama and Joyce drove me to the parking lot at Guilford.

I've already written about the transition to life at Guilford. I could never have dreamed, when I stepped out of the car that first day, less than two years later, I would be off on yet another leg of life's journey, as unprepared as I was for the preceding two years. Once again, I was in a new town – a much bigger city than I had spent seventeen years of my life learning to navigate, both geographically and socially. There were fresh faces, new schedules, new financial challenges – way too much "new" in my life. The only constant I had to hold onto was the Quaker meeting and Willie Frye.

In reviewing my text for these two years, I was struck by two glaring omissions: no mention of my family or, for that matter, anything or anybody outside my work at the hospital. Looking back at previous entries, I am stunned to see how little I have said about my family. I suppose that is true. However, in the fifty years Becky and I have been married, only twice have any of my siblings or cousins come to visit us in Kernersville (my sister Marlene (Faye). I have not been much better at keeping up the connections. Over all these years, I have driven to Goldsboro to attend nearly every annual family get-together. When Mama was still alive, I would visit her occasionally during the year. If I must be honest, I must realize when I left Goldsboro for Guilford College, I left Goldsboro!

I am saddened by the fact I have had so little to say about my family, especially Mama. I must give this some thought. I don't know where to go with that. What does this mean? Am I reading more into this omission than is warranted? The simple fact is my life, after dropping/flunking out of Guilford College, was consumed with dealing with the weight of that failure and disappointment, and the insecurity in not knowing what lay ahead after my CO obligation was completed. Failure and uncertainty are powerful obstacles to overcome! But, as these two years were ending, there was an unexpected Glimmer of Hope.

Chapter 11

HOPE ON THE HORIZON

IT'S THE SUMMER of 1971, and the world suddenly looks a little more enticing. After dating for only four months, this remarkable young woman has agreed to be my wife. I must say this. If either of my children had come home one evening and told me they were getting married after dating someone for only four months (and had not known this person very well at all before that), I would have told them they were nuts and they were not going to do such a thing. I probably would have thought that before Becky came into my life. Since then, with matters across the board, including my wife and children, I have learned to pause and think before reacting. Unfortunately, I'm not always successful at that. However, I always return to those four months that launched the path ahead.

During that summer, while finishing my obligation to Whitaker and preparing to return to Guilford in the fall, I reacquainted myself with another aspect of growing up. I re-discovered tobacco farming. I told friends when I graduated from high school and headed off to college, I was more excited about never again having to enter a cold, wet, rain-soaked tobacco field after a night of steady rain than I was about the prospects of what college might offer. I would never have to spend hours in a baking sun, surrounded by sticky, green leaves and who knows what crawling around at my feet. That may be a little hyperbole, but, at that point, not much. And now, what have I done? I have fallen crazy in love with the farmer's daughter. What am I going to do? They know I've worked in tobacco all my growing-up years. I messed up and told them. They didn't ask, but I had to offer to help.

I needed the points. This is a typical Southern generational farm family. And I'm a college dropout hospital orderly "draft dodger" who shows up to date their daughter. I'm sporting hair a little on the long side and a Mitch Miller goatee (look it up), shoes with heels an inch high, and wearing a men's bell bottom pants walking suit with vest, both striped like Joseph's coat of many colors. Like I said, I needed the points. So, after work and on days off, as needed, I would help the family and other hired help "put in tobacco." That's an expression that means help them harvest tobacco leaves, get them to the barn, and process them into the barn for heat curing. I would also help top and sucker the plants, help move irrigation pipes sometimes, and help remove cured tobacco from the barns and get it to the packhouse so Becky's mom and dad could organize and sort it before taking it to the warehouse for sale.

Tobacco farming was a hard way to make a living—a whole lot of hard, dirty work for a modest return. I never heard Peggy or Royce complain. In addition to tobacco, Royce maintained a herd of several dozen cattle for which he had to mow and bale hay for winter. I helped collect baled hay and get it to the barn. I even volunteered to ride the mower to mow their yard. They had more important things to do, and I didn't mind. I enjoyed the hay business. It kind of felt good to work and sweat.

I can't remember when, but Peggy took on a second job outside her farming duties somewhere along the way. Some nights and off days, she would paint. She had all the work she wanted, painting people's houses. Peggy was a strong woman who knew how something should be done. You knew it would be done right if you hired her to do something. Some years later, while they were still farming, and then continuing after they retired, Peggy worked part-time for Nestles. She was the salesperson who called on C-stores, ensuring they maintained sufficient inventory. Peggy was quite the sales rep. Over several years she was a star performer. Becky has heard me tell friends I have seen Peggy come in from a day's work in tobacco, go into the house, and come out thirty minutes later dressed for a sales call. You would never know she had spent all day in the hot sun hoeing, putting in tobacco, or working in a big family garden (and I do mean BIG). Then, as if by magic, she would emerge looking like some senior Corporate exec on her way to a board meeting- an amazing woman!

Lest I not give Becky's daddy equal time, let me say this. In over four decades of being around Royce and some of that working around him, I never, ever saw him lose his patience and utter a foul word to anyone. Operating a small family farm can tax a man's patience. Between the weather and the unreliable nature of temporary labor, getting a tobacco crop to the warehouse can get the best of a man. Never saw that happen with Royce. Add to that the unpredictable nature of a herd of cows and trying to keep them well-fed and fenced and where they are supposed to be when they are supposed to be there; well, it has gotten the better of many a good man. I never saw Royce lose his temper. I have memories of hearing him mutter a "rakafrat" under his breath a time or two. Now and then, I might overhear a "shoe box" so as not to let another "sh" utterance come out.

I came to love Royce and Peggy. After they realized their daughter was going to marry me, they opened wide their home and their hearts. Becky likes to say I got her mom's approval early because she liked how I ate. I was always invited to Sunday lunch after Becky, and I had been to church together at the Quaker meeting. I loved it. I felt right at home. It was always some combination of a traditional southern farm family Sunday lunch- fried chicken, meatloaf, turkey or ham, green beans, corn, mashed potatoes, rice, cornbread or rolls, and sweet tea. What was not to like? The problem was the rest of the family was a little picky in their eating habits. Not me! I jumped right in. It reminded me of many a family or family reunion meal back home. Becky says her mother liked to see me eat. I liked to eat. So, it all worked out well. Peggy and Royce were quite different personalities. Royce was the quiet, mischievous one. Peggy was the more outspoken, opinionated one. Becky says she has no idea how many times Royce had to kick Peggy under the table during some of those family Sunday lunches. Peggy was the go-getter in the pair. Royce was the plodder, the hang in there and get it done partner. He had that sheepish grin about him. I loved it.

I've rambled a little here. Suffice it to say the time from Becky saying "yes" on July 4th, 1971, to saying "I do" on June 18th, 1972, went by in a flash. It didn't feel that way at the time. We did get to know each other better. I continued my association with the Quaker meeting in Winston. She attended there with me. She had grown up attending Sedge Garden United Methodist Church near Kernersville. But she was willing to join me in the Quaker meeting. I appreciated that. I joined Becky and her family on a vacation camping trip to Myrtle

Beach, along with nearly a dozen other families, all from the Sedge Garden community and members of their church.

I returned to Guilford, driving from Winston to the campus four days a week. It was a challenging year in one regard. I could not afford to leave my job at Whitaker and go back to school without some source of support aside from financial aid. The hospital was good enough to hire me as an orderly part-time. I had to work nights and weekends on the regular hospital med-surge floors. It was different than my Whitaker experience. At Whitaker, I got to know the staff and patients. It was more like a family. That year in the general hospital, while trying to get back into a more successful academic routine and spend time with Becky, was challenging. It was just a job to go to. It wasn't a family. There were no Stans or Larrys. Becky understood. After all, she was in nursing school and understood hospital work's shifting nature. Some weeks I would get off work at 7:00 a.m. and get to class at Guilford just in time for Richie Zweigenhaft's 8:00 a.m. psychology class. I plugged along.

We survived. We did have some wonderful times together. Neither of us had any money, so we found less expensive venues. I bought a seasonal student pass for Tanglewood Park. We would go there to picnic and make out on a blanket. We would watch her brother Stan, two years younger than Becky, play baseball. Stan would follow us to Guilford. He became the starting catcher for Coach Stuart Maynard, setting school records for hitting. He was inducted into the Guilford College Sports Hall of Fame some years later. We enjoyed the movies. Becky competed in the Miss Winston-Salem pageant. Although she didn't win, she did win the best talent award. She did a terrific rendition of "I Have Confidence" from The Sound of Music. Julie Andrews had nothing on her.

The year went by, and we were primed to marry the next June. I must tell this story before moving on, back to before I proposed to Becky. I was in love with that girl from the first time I saw her. After we had dated for a while, I asked her to go with me to Goldsboro to meet my mother and maybe some of my family. And so we did. I had taken other girls to Goldsboro; not many, but some. This time was different. We made the trip, had a good weekend, and returned to Winston. A few weeks later, I made a solo trip back home. I had decided I was going to propose. Even though we had been dating less than four months by then, I had a good indication she might say "yes," as bizarre as that might seem. So, I went to Goldsboro to buy the tiniest little diamond ring you've ever seen. It was all I could afford. I was embarrassed by the size of it, not so much that I wouldn't go through with it. I was motivated.

I arrived in Goldsboro on a Friday afternoon, planning to go downtown on Saturday and find a ring. And that I did. Then, on Saturday night, I had to tell my mother what I was going to do, including going back to school. So, it was a lovely mid-summer evening, and Mama and I were sitting on the apartment's front porch. Mama was sitting in one of those metal chairs, popular in the sixties and seventies, green and white with little square-holed patterns. I was sitting beside her in the couch-like glider that was part of the set. We had been on the porch for a while, enjoying the evening air. I'm trying to get the courage to tell her what I was about to do. I couldn't get to the point. I was describing how much I liked this girl- "really liked"- what was I thinking? I told her about Becky's family and how they welcomed me. I told her how smart Becky was and what she was interested in regarding her nursing career. I was going on and on and getting nowhere. Finally, My mama stopped me in my tracks and asked, and I am quoting here because I will remember her question until the day I die; She stopped me in midsentence and asked, "Gene, you ain't in no trouble, are you?" She caught me totally by surprise. I blurted out, "No! No! I'm going to ask her to marry me." From then on, it was all downhill. I told her my trip downtown earlier in the day was to buy a ring. I showed it to her. I told her I had fallen in love the minute I met her. I realized we had only been dating for four months, but I knew this was the one. I told her I never imagined getting married before finishing college, but if Becky said yes, we would figure it out. It was all OK from then on. Mama liked Becky when she visited. She liked that she came from a farm family. The next day I returned to Winston- a man on a mission.

Hope and Horizons! What an appropriate juxtaposition of concepts. Midway through my self-imposed two-year exile away from academia, I had all but lost all hope. My life was far removed from the dreams I had visualized just a couple of short years earlier. I remember Bud and me working in the summer and talking about the future. I could see myself becoming a trustee of Guilford College one day, maybe even its President. Talk about Hope! How absurd! Life can do that, you know. It can play tricks on you. In one moment, circumstances can coalesce to conjure up all kinds of improbable missions, experiences, and even outcomes. A poor, painfully shy, introverted first-generation college kid from The Project could become the President of

such a place as Guilford College. When flirting with such Hope, I had no idea what was involved in actualizing such a thing. Life has a not-so-funny way of getting in the way of Hope sometimes.

For Hope to have any real meaning and potential for finding a place in reality, there must be at least one Horizon that can be seen; and if not seen, at least visualized in such a manner that it becomes "real." Like Hope, Horizons can play cruel jokes on the unsuspecting or naïve believer. How does one, caught up in their moment of Hope, distinguish between a Horizon that personifies all that Hope promises and its deceitful counterimage- a dry, barren, lifeless mirage? I don't know. I do know life can be filled with these conflicting moments. I also know it can be difficult, if not impossible, to realize this core fact in real-time. By its very nature, Hope assumes a level of trust, belief, and imagination that allows every Horizon to be attainable, even if it was never real in the first place. On the other hand, who gets to decide when a Horizon is real and achievable or when it is only a dry, barren mirage where a life-giving oasis stood only moments before?

There's that question again. Who gets to decide? We've paused on that one before. Who gets to determine if a Horizon is real or not? What kind of Hope factors into this dynamic? Can Hope bring to life a dry, barren mirage? Or, are there genetic and socio-cultural limitations that Hope can only flirt with in the margins? The ledger is full of those one-in-a-million stories where indescribable Hope and unimaginable Horizons coalesce. The question that drives the plot for me is who decides who manages to get that one-in-a-million straw. What separates that storyline from others who fail to experience the meshing of their Hopes and Horizons?

Maybe someday???

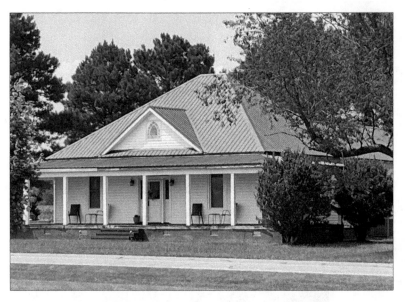

Old Homeplace- site of Hurricane Hazel photo 2023

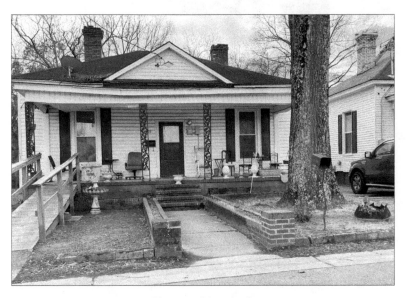

House on Chestnut St

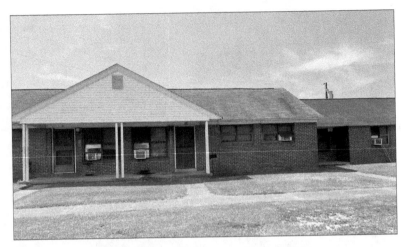

Fairview Homes (The Project)- photo 2023

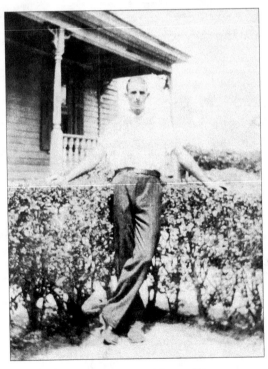

Daddy, only photo I have of him

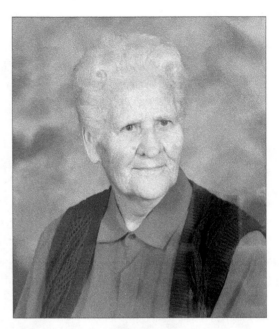

Mama

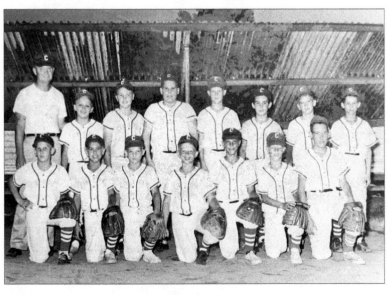

Little League Civitans 1959

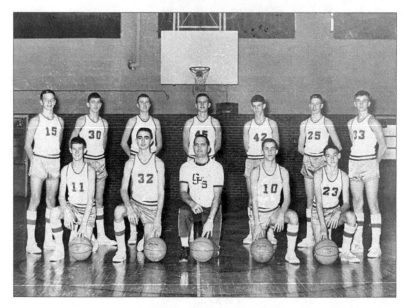

7th & 8th grade basketball team

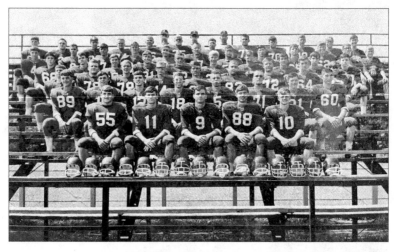

Football Team 1966 (Gohisca Yearbook)

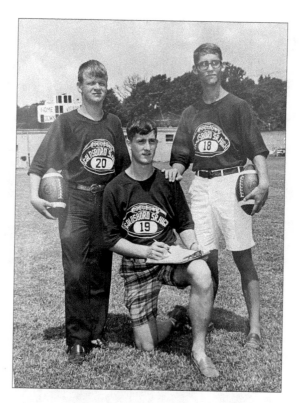

Optimist Oratorical Contestants with Coach Whis (Goldsboro News-Argus)

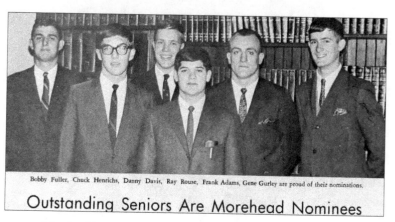

Bobby Fuller, Chuck Henrichs, Danny Davis, Ray Rouse, Frank Adams, Gene Gurley are proud of their nominations.

Outstanding Seniors Are Morehead Nominees

Morehead Scholarship nominees, 1967 (Goldsboro News-Argus)

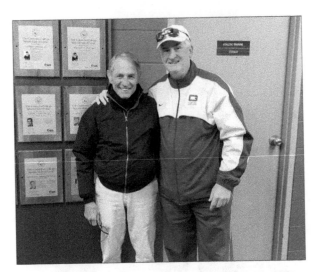

Coach Whis and me, 2017 during our visit to The Hill

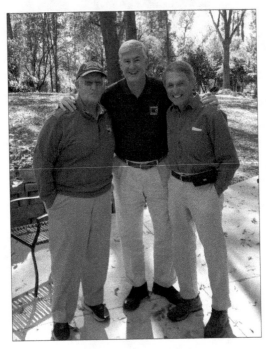

Coaches Whisenhunt and Whitfield, 2017 during that same trip

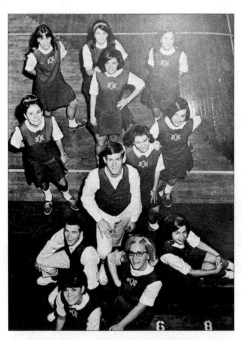

Guilford College cheerleading squad, 1969
(Guilford College QUAKER Yearbook)

Guilford academic transcript. Part 1– nothing to be proud of

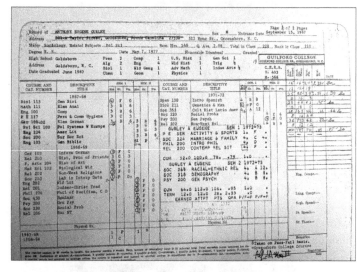

Guilford academic transcript. Part 2- proof that hope springs eternal

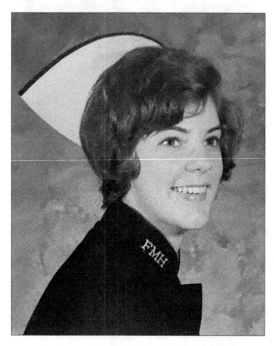

Cutest student nurse ever, 1971, still is

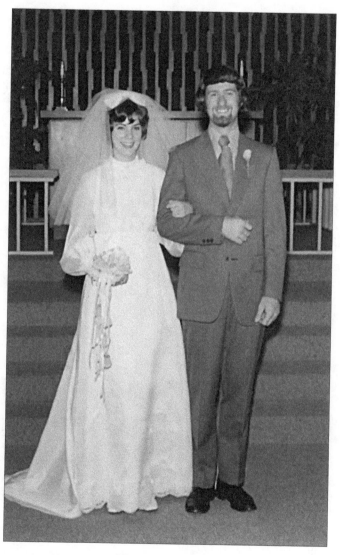

Wedding Day, 1972

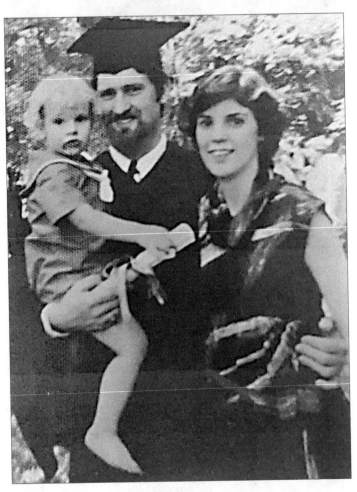

Guilford graduation, 1972

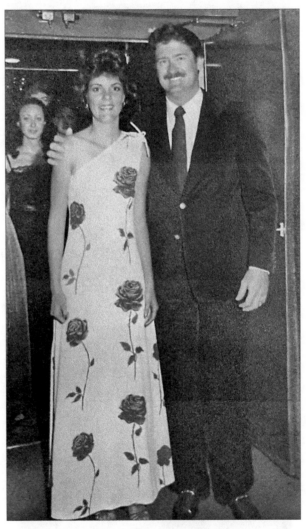

10ᵗʰ-anniversary cruise, 1982

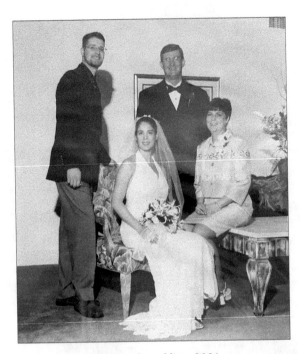

Daughter's wedding, 2001

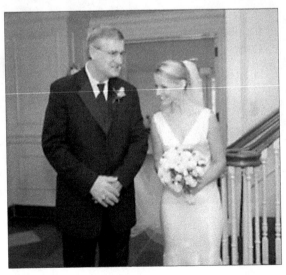

DeAnn's wedding day

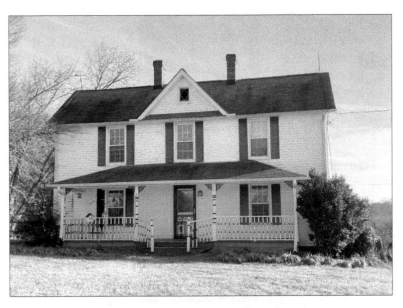

Old farmhouse, home since 1985, four generations

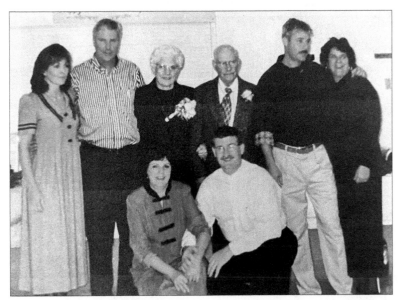

Peggy & Royce's 60th anniversary, with Becky's brothers and their wives

181

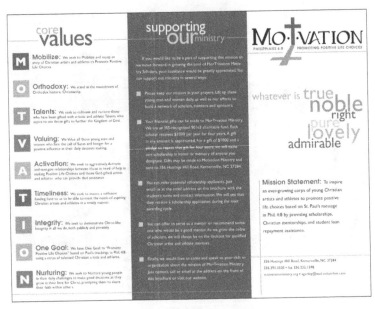

Motvation Ministry brochure

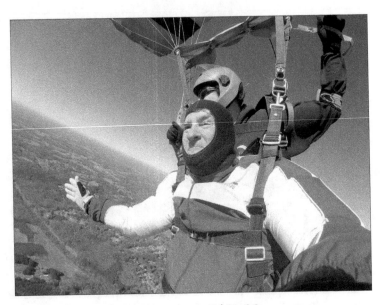

Skydiving on my 69th birthday

182

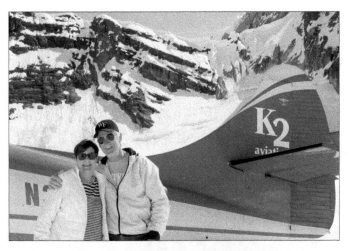

50th–anniversary road trip through Alaska

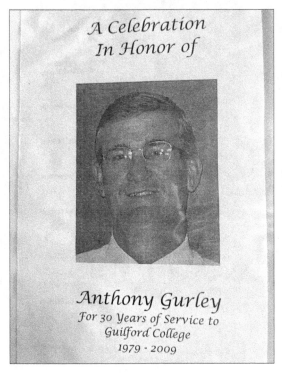

A Celebration
In Honor of

Anthony Gurley
For 30 Years of Service to
Guilford College
1979 - 2009

Retirement from Guilford College to launch Motvation Ministry

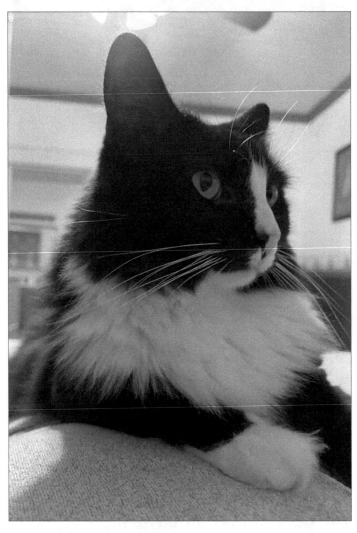

Jethro, *My Buddy*

Chapter 12

STARTING A NEW LIFE TOGETHER

I COULDN'T WAIT to get back to Winston-Salem. I knew what I was going to do. I didn't know some of the formalities that go along with this process. I didn't know I was supposed to get the intended father's permission to ask his daughter to marry me. Such formalities were outside the scope of my upbringing. All I knew was next week was the 4th of July, and that is when it would happen. I had arranged with the Selective Service to cut my 2-year obligation short by a few weeks to return to college in mid-August. I had applied for readmission to Guilford, and they had said "yes." So, to cap off a terrific summer, I was going to "pop the question" on July 4th at one of Stan's American Legion baseball games. How romantic is that? Some fifty-one years later, I can't recall how I was so sure Becky would say "yes." After all, we had been dating only four months. Somehow, I knew. I just knew. So, that's what I did. She said "yes" and did so with one of her heart-melting smiles. I don't know if I have ever had a happier moment in my life. She hugged and kissed me in a way that told me she really did love me in a way I had never felt before. A year later, on June 18th, 1972, that "yes" became an "I do." I still wonder how such a beautiful, bright, and talented young Godly woman falls in love with and says "yes" to marriage after just four months of dating a college dropout with no family financial backing and an unknown future. I have only one answer to that question- it must be a "God thing." I have many questions about God and how it all works. I do not question God's existence. I have spent a good portion of my life in arenas where that accepted existence is part and parcel of the culture of those arenas. I still do not understand the hows or the whys of that existence. All I do know is in that moment on the evening of July 4th, in the parking lot of a small-town American Legion Baseball game, God showed up. Nothing in my life is more clear to me than that. There have been other such "God moments" over the years. There have also been moments (and episodes) outside our marriage when I found myself asking where God was or why did the same God who produced that beautiful moment now leave me in such a state of isolation and failure.

Since I had failed to follow the proper protocol for getting permission, Becky and I had some news to share with her parents. We drove straight to her house and waited in the kitchen for her mom and dad to arrive. They had been at the same game we attended. They never missed one of Stan's games. They arrived after what seemed like hours (quite sure it was less than 40 minutes). I can't recall how we told them, but we did. I don't recall any particular emotional response. I'm pretty sure they were surprised, perhaps shocked, maybe even disappointed. Knowing their daughter the way I do, I doubt they harbored the same question my mama did (You're not in any trouble, are you?) I am sure they had not expected this news at this point in their daughter's life. I did not know this then, but Becky had been in a committed relationship when we had our first date. It's easy to see how her parents might have still thought that relationship was still in play.

There we were Royce, Peggy, Becky, and me- standing in the kitchen, digesting the news. I don't remember Becky's dad saying anything. Over the years, I learned he was a man of few words. Peggy did the talking. The first response came from her. She asked if we were planning a December wedding when Becky would be on Christmas break from nursing school. She had one more year of school. We told her, "No." We would wait until Becky finished school. We told them I was going back to Guilford in the fall, and it just made sense to wait for one of us to finish school. That settled the matter for the time being. I drove back to my room.

I have no idea what conversations ensued that night after my departure or on future occasions when Becky was at home. What I do know is this- Becky's parents have never treated me with anything other than respect and love. I have told many folks Becky's father, Royce, in many ways, became the father I never had. I loved that man dearly. I have none of the mechanical skills or problem-solving acumen that Royce possessed. He never once let that get in the way of our relationship. I felt nothing when I received the news years ago that my dad had passed. It was not so when Royce died. I miss him.

Overall, the ensuing year was a great time. I did not particularly like my job at the hospital. But it paid the bills- just barely- and provided enough for an occasional movie or trip to Mayberry's Ice Cream Shop. I enjoyed getting to know a couple of Becky's classmates, and we would occasionally do things together. Getting back into school was a challenge. I was commuting from Winston-Salem and trying to get to Guilford for eight o'clock classes after working the third shift at the hospital. I was eager to be the kind of student I knew I could be, the kind Becky would be proud of. It was hard. Money was an issue. It always has been. I was torn between wanting good grades, wanting to spend time with Becky, and having to work in a job and schedule I hated. I remember finding myself occasionally, during quiet times in the hospital during the wee hours of the morning, or in the car trying to stay awake to drive to Guilford, thinking, why does this have to be so complicated? This may seem like the petty self-pitying of an old man, considering so much that is just wrong in the world today. Maybe it was. It could be. I was always so elated every minute I was in Becky's presence, only to find myself sinking back into an emotional abyss that seemed (seems?) to have no end. There was/is no end to the self-flagellation that takes me far away from that joy. It does no good to try not to think about my life compared to those I see and wonder why them and not me. It usually comes down to a material comparison. I know I have been blessed with a wonderful wife and terrific offspring. For that, I am grateful. Why couldn't I have that AND be more professionally and financially successful? People say- "you don't know what 'they' have going on in their lives. You don't know what struggles 'they' have experienced." I get that. This tendency to compare my life and experiences unfavorably to others while I have only a distant and vague view of their realities has always plagued me. Now, in retirement, I wake each day and consciously realize life will never be any better; that today is probably as good as it will ever be. I cannot get away from the nagging reminders of how I have fallen so short of the potential I had. Now, those opportunities are forever gone. Unrealized opportunities can never become invigorating memories.

That year passed quickly. Becky was a super student, as she has always been. On the other hand, I still did not live up to my potential. I did manage to move in the right direction. Proper motivation and focus were still lacking. The spring of 1972 approached, and the wedding day was coming. We knew we wanted a church wedding. We were married in the sanctuary at Sedge Garden United Methodist Church, where Becky had grown up, and her mother was an active leader, later becoming a Trustee, to be followed as such by her daughter a few decades later. The wedding was beautiful and simple. As money was scarce, the men wore suits rather than tuxes. The ceremony was officiated by Rev. Leon Stubbs, the senior pastor at the church and a longtime family friend of Becky and her family. Becky and her brothers had grown through their teen years with the Reverend's children. The second pastor officiating was Willie Frye, my friend, and mentor at Winston-Salem Friends Meeting. Becky and I wrote our vows. Those vows, translated into Japanese, now hang beside each other in our living room. (Becky has long loved Asian art. I was able to have the wife of a Guilford professor translate the vows for me. I had them framed and given to Becky as an anniversary gift many years ago).

Becky's family was a mainstay in the church. She had been regularly active. In her teenage years and into her time in nursing school, she participated in a Lay Witness domestic mission program. She and her family were loved by all. As a result, when the wedding day came, the place was filled. I can only imagine what must have gone through the minds of many of her family and longtime friends and acquaintances. What in the world was she doing? I also had a good portion of my family from Goldsboro in attendance. My oldest nephew Jerry (only four years younger than me) spent the night before the wedding with me in my room at the house right across the street from the Quaker meetinghouse. Jerry still talks about that night, listening to me, trying to make sure I had memorized my vows. Standing in front of a full church the next day and choking on my lines would be embarrassing. He helped, and I did fine the following afternoon.

Keeping with the low-budget theme Becky and I left the wedding reception in the church fellowship hall and managed to elude our pursuers, who were intent on "decorating" my car. I had reserved a week in an apartment on the banks of a gently flowing creek on the outskirts of Gatlinburg, TN. Gatlinburg has always been a popular honeymoon venue. We both agreed it would be a good destination if we didn't get too caught up in the tourist-ism. We found the right place to get out, see the sights, and have the privacy and seclusion we wanted. It was beautiful. At night, we could leave the sliding door to the screen open and hear the water rushing by. We had a wonderful week-all that a honeymoon should be. Then, we returned to the Triad and moved into our Frazier apartment on the Guilford Campus. I continued my classes, and Becky got a job at Wesley Long Hospital in labor & delivery, her first-choice nursing specialty. Even though I struggled to return to school, life looked good.

The following two years were an emotional roller coaster for me. I don't know how much of that ride Becky experienced. Becky tends to keep things "bottled up." Where my two semesters back at Guilford had not been stellar, I was passing most of my work with A's and B's. My first semester after our wedding, in the fall of 1972, my grades went to Hell in a hand-basket again. I flunked two of the four courses I took. One was a 1-credit hour PE activity course. How do you do that? I didn't show up for class- a failing pattern is beginning to emerge again. I managed to get it together before the spring semester, and I made two A's and a B. Still not what I was capable of doing, but it was a re-start in the right direction. Or so I thought. I decided to go to summer school to make up for some lost credits. I wasn't all that interested in schoolwork. I just wanted to make better grades and graduate- sooner rather than later. With the number of failed courses on my transcript, it would take a bit to make all that up. So, summer school in the summer of 1973 it was. And, what d'ya know? I made three A's and two B's. I was back on track.

We bought a registered dachshund puppy and named him Fritz; Fritz von Rasputin was his official registered name. That was a dream come true for me. All my years growing up in The Project, we could not have pets. I had always wanted a dog. Becky and I saw Fritz at a venue at the Guilford County Fair. I fell in love, and I think Becky was happy about it too. She had always been around dogs. Royce raised, trained, and competed fox hounds. We took Fritz home, and he became a focal point in our young family- in violation of college policy about pets in the apartments.

But something wasn't right. That albatross I had carried for years continued to find its way back. Becky was working hard and enjoying her job. I worked part-time- loading trucks on weekends at Pilot Freight. I got a morning paper route where I had to drive to cover the size of the route. We didn't live extravagantly. We never had enough money to cover things. I began to build up credit card debt. I would bounce checks. Once again, I was embarrassed. Once again, I just wanted it all to stop. And, once again, stop it did; or, stop, I did. By the fall of 1973, just a year after our wedding, I again began reverting to sluffing off schoolwork, avoiding classes, and working to make ends meet. That fall, I failed half my classes. The following spring, I essentially quit being a student again. I got a full-time job with NCNB-North Carolina National Bank (predecessor to Bank of America). By then, it was too late to withdraw without failing grades, so my transcript shows I flunked the three courses I "took."

Part of the real tragedy of all this is I hid it so well. At least, I think I did. I don't know to what extent Becky was aware of how poorly I was doing academically and emotionally. I was good at camouflaging it. I got a decent job and was ready to quit school again and work to support my family. At least, that's how I remember presenting it. I didn't need a degree to work at the bank. It never occurred at the front end of the process; I was going nowhere without a degree. Quit school again. Call people to get them to pay their bills (the irony of this now fifty-one years later is mind-boggling) and repossess cars, boats, and mobile homes- that was going to be my path to life as a successful banker. Life would be good. How stupid could I have been?

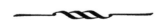

What is a God-thing"? A God moment? We often hear of someone who has experienced a 'miraculous' event- a financial windfall, a recovery from illness, or an escape from a life-shattering accident. Perhaps we have experienced such ourselves. As Believers, we often attribute these outcomes to the intervention of God- "a God thing." We hear the acclamation "God is Good" when we hear or see these miraculous occurrences. Do we hear this exclamation when we learn one of our students has been diagnosed with colon cancer? Where is the God-thing when a sick twenty-year-old walks into the school building and leaves a dozen or more families in a state of untold remorse, anger, and

emptiness? Why are we quick to ascribe credit and give thanks for the intervention of God on the one hand and remain silent when it appears God chooses to remain on the sidelines?

The roots of most of the failures, disappointments, and shortcomings recounted in this exercise can be laid at the feet of the writer. There! That said, how does a player in this drama come to terms with an effort to Believe in that Presence and give it proper credit when those God-moments occur, and at the same time, accept personal responsibility for all those other minutes, hours, days when that Presence is hard to recognize? Amid this ever-recurring lapse into a failing behavior, the question beckons, "Why does it have to be so hard?"

Hard is a relative term. Could it be that, in relative terms, the life unfolding in these pages in no way qualifies as a "hard "one? The writer has been loved, has never suffered any serious illness or physical injury, and was born and raised in the most wealthy and free place in the world. Life has been one with opportunities for a level of success and happiness that is unknown to much of the rest of humankind. The problem is no one lives their life in relative terms. Life is lived in real, personal, in-the-moment definitive terms. So, I believe the question, "Why does it have to be so hard?" is a fair one. I believe trying to understand the continuum between God's Presence and the absence of the intervention of that Presence, all in the name of freedom to choose, is a valid internal struggle.

These years that encompassed the start of a new life together were the manifestation of that dichotomy. Now, all these years later, I still struggle with that dichotomy. Life has had its share of those God-moments. For that, I am grateful. But life has also been too full of that same failure to seize the moment, take advantage of the opportunities, ask for help, and believe my opinion and efforts are just as valuable as the next guy's. Now, I don't know if this matters much anymore other than as intellectual and theological calisthenics. It may have mattered once upon a time.

All I know is I am a fortunate man that the woman I love more than life itself chose not to ever give up on me. Subsequent years have not been devoid of these failings and changes in direction. Was our recent 50ᵗʰ-anniversary evidence of a fulfilled promise, a God-thing? Or, is it simply a logical result of fifty years of peaks and valleys, successes and failures, of Hopes fostered and real or imagined Horizons? Or- is there some interconnectedness in this mosaic I cannot understand? When does the cost of waging the battle become too steep? When is it time to surrender to the struggle or decide emphatically that the answer is unimportant? Is one to just go on living life, with or without the Presence, and with or without any understanding of why any of this matters?

Chapter 13

WILL I NEVER LEARN?

NO LONGER A student, we had to vacate the student's apartment. Working at the bank and with Becky's income from the hospital, we were able to buy our first house. It just goes to show how easy home buying was in those days. No respectful banker should have loaned us that money. We moved into our little house on Marion Street in Greensboro and started down our new path. Once again, life was going to be wonderful. But no! My whole life has consisted of stumbling mindlessly down one path to nowhere, only to get sidetracked onto another. We did make some good friends at work then. We were in a constant state of flux. Not long after we moved to Marion St., the bank decided to restructure its consumer credit calling program. I had the choice of losing my job or moving to Durham to continue to work the caseload I had been working from the center in Greensboro. Neither Becky nor I had planned on this. Neither of us had ever talked about leaving the Triad area. I had started down this road, and we seemed to have no choice.

Looking back, I know this development was disappointing to Becky. She never complained. We had to sell the house we had just bought and find something to rent in Durham. You know where this is leading-more debt. Looking back on that time, I marvel at how Becky handled it. It may have been better had she said no, I won't go. I don't know how that might have changed the course of our lives. As this story unfolds, I hope one thing is clear. No matter the failures before and after Becky came into my life, the disappointments, the shortcomings when I compare myself to others—whatever has led me to this dilemma, let me be *very clear*, none of the blame for this rests on Becky's shoulders. If anything, this journey would likely have reached this crossroads long before now had it not been for her love and faithfulness to our union. Without going down another rabbit hole now, know she has been and is my anchor. Even in those recurring, fleeting moments when I find myself doubting God's plan or even his Presence, I never doubt Becky's rock-solid foundation. She is a fantastic woman. She deserved better.

We moved to Durham and rented a nice house in a suburb north of town. By this time, we had added another dachshund to the family- Gretchen. Becky got a job at the old Watts Hospital in Durham. The facility and grounds would later become the NC School of Math and Science. We were back on schedule. Oh- I forgot to mention. Before leaving Greensboro, we learned we were going to become parents. Becky was pregnant with our first child. We were not trying to get pregnant. We were taking precautions. We could not afford a baby. (Can you ever?) But most of all, I was terrified of the prospect of becoming a father. I had no idea how to be a father. I had visceral memories of the few years with my father. Those memories, such as they were, were not good. Pretty much all I learned from him was to stay out of his way and "don't ask for a damn thing." I have few memories of time spent with him other than a couple of miserable fishing trips to Blounts Creek north of New Bern. He scared me to death with eels and kept telling me to be still and shut up. How could you catch any fish with such commotion in the little John boat we were in? I remember my brother Buddy going with us. He and Daddy seemed to get along fine. I was very much "in the way." Thinking back, the only reason I went on either of those trips was because Mama insisted on it. I also remember him and Mama taking me out of school one day so I could accompany him as he delivered a prisoner to the state prison in Raleigh. That was one of his many duties as a guard at the local prison farm. I must have been in the fourth or fifth grade. I think he was trying to scare me. It worked. I can still see the halls and hear the metal doors closing.

At any rate, I was horrified at the prospect of becoming a daddy. I knew I had no real physical skills to pass along to a child. As time grew closer to the due date and we knew we would have a son, I panicked. I didn't know anything about how to raise a son. I couldn't teach him anything that, at least back in those days, culture thought little boys should learn. I am mechanically inept. The news of an unexpected baby, when we were in the midst of so much continuing failure on my part and disruption in our lives, was not welcome news. Once again, I felt useless and not in control of anything in my life. I was not happy.

I found my place at work in the Foster Street branch of the bank where the Consumer Credit Dept. was located. I made friends, only one of whom I would stay in touch with after that brief stint in Durham. After Scot was born, I enjoyed meeting Becky for lunch on her days off. She would bring Scot, and I would meet them at a nearby mall. Those were good times. As unhappy as I had been with the news I would soon be a daddy, I was equally happy at the sight of our little boy. I loved him dearly, and Becky was such a terrific mom.

There was one scary episode not long before Scot was born. One of our neighbors worked in an animal research lab at Duke University. They had brought home a coyote and kept it in a pen in their backyard. By now, our first dachshund had been killed, run over by a car while visiting Becky's parents, but not before breeding with Gretchen. Gretchen was pregnant and just a short time away from birthing her puppies. Becky was near term also. One afternoon while I was at work, Becky was on the small back patio when this coyote showed up in the yard. Gretchen immediately went into protection mode. Becky grabbed a broom and commenced trying to run off the coyote. So here is my pregnant wife and our pregnant dachshund trying to protect each other. Becky managed to run it off, but not before it attacked Gretchen. Becky took her to a local vet, and I met them there. The doctor was not able to save Gretchen. He was able to deliver three puppies that survived. What happened next is one of the most amazing things I have ever witnessed.

We have three newborn dachshund puppies we now need to feed and raise to a point where we can find homes for them. We tried baby bottles with the formula the vet suggested. It was not working well. I remember hearing Becky tell stories about one of the dogs they had at their home in Kernersville. Royce had raised and competed with hunting dogs for many years. They also had other dogs around the farm. Becky told me about one of those dogs, Cricket, which was on the farm at the time. Becky had seen Crickett bring baby rabbits up to the house and commence to feed and care for them. We assume she found them in the woods or pastures surrounding the home. Perhaps their mother had been killed by a coyote or some other predator.

At any rate, Crickett nursed these little creatures to health. I do not begin to understand the ways of nature in this regard.

I believed that if Crickett could rescue a baby rabbit and her motherly instincts turn on such that she could produce milk sufficient to keep a baby rabbit alive, then she could do the same thing for three starving dachshund puppies. We drove to Kernersville and brought Crickett back to Durham. She immediately "took to" the puppies and began " mothering" them. Soon she began to produce milk. All three puppies survived, and we found great homes and families for them.

I tell this story to make a point I'm not sure I appreciated at the time. This was a traumatic experience. We loved Gretchen. Becky was in a very vulnerable state. Our lives together for such a short time had been full of directional changes and disappointments. During all that, we saw a miracle of nature take place. I don't know how all that stuff works. I know what I saw. Occasionally, over the years, I have thought back on that 'miracle' and wondered why I have not seen more of that kind of miraculous outcome. I don't know. Have they occurred, and I have too blind to see them? Or are they not miracles at all-none of them? Is life such that sometimes stuff just happens and sometimes it doesn't?

Scot was born on June 20th, 1975, at Watts Hospital. I continued my work at NCNB, calling to collect past-due payments and going out to repossess cars and such. I can't say repossessing someone's car or truck was fun. Often, by the time it came to that, I had called and been lied to so many times I didn't care what kind of disadvantage taking the vehicle created for the customer or what they thought of me and my heritage.

Scot's arrival was impactful in many ways. Some are the obvious ones, lack of sleep and increased bills. No more just getting in the car to go somewhere. Now it was a production to take a trip- out for the evening or back to grandma and grandpa in Kernersville or granny in Goldsboro. In a few months, I began feeling the urge to change directions again. If there is anything consistent in this story, it is that little has been consistent, dependable, or well-planned in my life. I don't know if that is anybody's fault. That's how it had been, at least up to that point. A few years later, a more consistent and reliable scenario would emerge. Even then, it would have its own underbelly of disappointment and failure.

I had been at the bank for less than two years. That was long enough to see I had no future with the organization if I didn't have at least an undergraduate degree. I could see all the branch managers and vice presidents had degrees. I could see the "fast trackers" come through; young, recent college graduates (or MBA grads). They rarely stayed long enough to break a sweat before going off to a branch. Even the staff in our office, those who were fixtures in that environment, all had degrees and were biding their time until they got a shot up the ladder in Corporate management- not necessarily in the branches. So, once again, I was about to impose on Becky and our new family another move and, of course, more unplanned change. Sitting here, reliving those days, I am seeing for the first time just how much disruption I foisted upon Becky. To my recollection, she never balked. I didn't fully appreciate how self-centered all this changing course and failing to follow through was. It did not occur to me how unfair I was being to Becky. Looking back, I don't know how she stayed with me. Sitting here at the beach writing, enjoying a one-week vacation before her fall semester at Rockingham Community College begins, I can see her working on her jewelry, something she loves to do. I interrupted her work momentarily to tell her where I am in this process, finishing this phase of the story. I told her I could not fathom how she could tolerate the ride those first few years. Her response- "I loved you."This is one of those peaks I wrote about in my letter.

We discussed it, and I decided. I was going back to college. This time I had a choice to make. Should I return to Guilford? Would they take me a third time? Or might I try to get into Chapel Hill? We could stay where we were or move into student apartments in Chapel Hill. I did some research and found the name of the person I needed to speak with at Chapel Hill. I had decided wherever I went, I would continue my pursuit of a degree in Sociology with a strong minor in Political Science. This was in 1975. The country was coming off a long and divisive war in Vietnam and was in what will continue to be a decades-long Civil Rights struggle. I made an appointment to meet with a professor whose name I cannot remember. He was head of the Peace Studies Program. UNC had done something a handful of universities around the country did. Rising from the anti-war sentiment across the country, there was a clarion call from the left to abolish all ROTC programs on college campuses. UNC opted not to do this. They retained the programs and put them under the control of the director of the Peace Studies Program. That is who I was to see. I cannot begin to cover all we talked about in that session. I do know it was life-altering.

When I left Guilford the second time, I was in a dark place-again. I had failed to succeed academically and could not adequately support my wife. When I flunked out of Guilford after two years, I convinced myself I failed because of the war and the civil unrest all around me. I've often used the excuse that with daily news reports about the war and the riots, the last place I needed to be was in an 8:00 a.m. English class talking about Beowulf. The professor I met that day in Chapel Hill kept emphasizing a case could be made that college dropouts/flunk outs during that period could easily be attributed to a mental state of unrest so profound that one could excuse that failure and extend additional opportunities to flourish. He made me feel so good, so positive about myself. I was not alone on the road I had traveled the past few years. He confirmed what I had been telling myself and others about why I had not made it at Guilford. He said there was a whole generation of young men like me; young men who had not gone off to war, whose lives had also been disrupted, and whose mental states were unhinged in different ways, but still emotionally degrading. He assured me UNC would look kindly upon my application. He could see to that. He also suggested Guilford, mainly due to its Quaker heritage, would likely give me another chance. After all, I had been working and doing well in a good job and had started a family. He knew enough about Guilford to be familiar with its Center for Continuing Education. He was confident they would let me back in.

The irony of that meeting was he reinforced a lie I had been telling myself and others since departing Guilford, even up to the writing of this epistle. English classes and Beowulf had nothing to do with my poor performance at Guilford- not the first time there, nor the second time. That was all a ruse to avoid the truth. I blew the first opportunity at Guilford because I couldn't live the life most of my friends lived. I wanted desperately to fit in and enjoy the experience. I could not bring myself to ask for help. When I did not understand a concept or a lab experience, I could not seek help from a professor or another student. Instead, I would hide irrationally, hoping it would all go away. That was sick. But that is the truth.

So, back to Guilford we went. I gave my notice at the bank, and Becky did so at Watts. We made a couple of day trips to Greensboro to find somewhere to live. Married student apartments at Guilford were not an option with a little one. Six months after Scot joined our family, we were off to start down, yet another road- one that had some considerable familiarity to it yet would develop in totally unexpected ways.

There's not much to reflect on here. A young couple, just beginning to figure out how to navigate married life, picks up and moves away from all they know and love because one-half the couple is adrift in a sea of uncertainty about life and his role in it. He is afraid of everything and petrified his better half will discover she has made a huge mistake. Neither of the players in this drama has any experience handling money. One of them never had any. The other grew up with parents who were not wealthy but were good stewards of what they did have, and she never wanted for anything of importance. Her parents built the house she grew up in with their own hands and never had a house payment. Other than a shared farm background (to some extent), they had so little in common from which to nurture their marriage. But, nurtured it was. Uh-oh! If I'm not careful, I'll be drifting back to that, was it "a God-thing" discussion? Not going there. I'm too tired of it all to give it fair measure.

Suffice it to come to the resolution that life is just way too full of unknowns. I'll never know why Daddy didn't try to keep me in his life after he walked out; other than to acknowledge he didn't make much of an effort to have me in it before he walked out. I'll never understand how Becky said "Yes" when she did and has continued to do so all these years. I'll never know why I couldn't rise above the fears that have shackled much of my life. Intellectually knowing something and acting on that knowledge are two very different things. Life could have been so much more stimulating, fulfilling, and productive if only knowledge could have always produced the rational actions one might assume knowledge has the power to do. It hasn't.

In many ways, these two years in Durham were a watershed period. The years following were filled with many of the same kinds of poor choices or choices that defaulted out of fear, which were at the core of life up to then. There was one significant difference. The time in Durham, and the arrival of Scot, did change things. Despite the shortcomings already mentioned, stability did center down upon our family after the arrival of Scot and the decision to return to college. Subsequent chapters will reveal some of this. There would still be bad choices, devouring fears, and missed opportunities. Something would be different. I don't know how much of a God-thing I can attribute it to.

As the reader will see later, I am still uncertain about God's role in all this. I know that post-Durham, our lives as a family did begin to have an element of structure and stability that had evaded us previously. This is not unique to our launch as a young couple. I am sure I didn't recognize it until it revealed itself during this exercise.

***Friends-Choices-Consequences!** As an old man now, I begin to see and appreciate the roles and interconnectedness of these three things. I wish I could have better recognized their worth and yielded myself to that recognition earlier in my life. I may have been able to address the fears that governed much of the years both before and after Durham.*

Chapter 14

GUILFORD COLLEGE 3.0

BECKY AND I quit our jobs before Christmas and moved back to Greensboro in time for the holidays. Scot was six months old. His addition to the family was a major motivating factor in my decision to return to school. We rented a two-bedroom house on Home Street near the Greensboro Coliseum. We were happy to be back "home," as it were. We enjoyed the holidays being close to Becky's family. I prepared for the start of the spring semester at Guilford. Becky readied herself to work at Wesley Long again, back in labor and delivery- where she felt wonderfully comfortable. We made the move back for all the right reasons. Deep inside, I was still burdened by the fear I would fail once again. This was my third strike. There would be no more.

We had the schedule all worked out. I got a morning paper route that helped with school and household expenses. I could be home in time to get to class and be done with classes by the time Becky went to the hospital for her 3-11 shift. When she went to work, I split my time between homework and looking after Scot. I have never been a morning person. I had to be up and out of bed by about 4:00 to get to my newspaper pick-up spot and get the papers rolled and delivered before 6:30. My route was on the north side of Greensboro, between downtown and Cone Hospital. I had a lot of hospital staff on my route. If they didn't get their paper before 6:30, they didn't need it. By the time they would get home from work, they were reading history, not news. So, I had to make that early morning delivery.

I would get home, change clothes (maybe), and get to campus. Fortunately, that was only about a ten-minute drive. We planned for me to graduate in the spring of 1977 after attending three semesters and a summer school. That plan left little room for extras or unnecessary sleep. I rarely went to bed before Becky got home around 11:30. I just liked being awake when she came in late at night. I did learn to nap during the day when Scot would. If I could nap a little during the day, I could get by with only 4 -4 ½ hours of sleep at night.

We plowed right into the first semester and the new jobs. I had no idea if this was going to work. Then, something miraculous happened. Despite the lack of sleep, the tight schedules, and trying to be a good father and husband, I had pulled all A's by the end of that first semester. I only took 12 hours that first semester and summer school, but I was determined to give myself a chance. I aced all three classes in the spring and again in summer school. I began to believe! I began to feel a weight being lifted. I was proving to myself I could succeed, a feeling long departed from my psyche. Becky was immensely supportive. And, one of the unexpected long-term benefits began to emerge. As stated earlier, the schedule called for me to be home with Scot after Becky went to work. That meant I was the one to look after him during his waking hours from mid-afternoon till bedtime. Sometimes that was exhausting. After having been awake myself since 4:00 in the morning, it was my duty to stay awake with him when he was awake, feed him on time, bathe him, and put him to bed. Sometimes it all went like clockwork. Sometimes, it was a challenge. Sometimes, when his bedtime came, I was in such a state that neither of us handled it well. We both survived. Ah, but that long-term benefit.

Scot is now 47 years old, and his pappy is 73. I'm not sure when I realized it; at some point, I did. Those hours together at that point in our lives were a tremendous blessing most fathers do not experience. Few fathers get to be their child's primary caregiver during half their waking hours regularly. Few fathers get to be the ones responsible for putting their children to bed and reading them bedtime stories on a regular basis. As the years have wandered by, I have thought about that year and a half a lot. I know I did not appreciate it then. Given my lack of a relationship with my father, and my fear of becoming a father when I first heard the news, I had no reason to anticipate the upside of that experience. Over the years, I have grown to know just how special that time was.

Scot and I are quite different in many ways. He is a talented artist and a more voracious reader than I am. He has never had much of an interest in sports. Like me, Scot tends to be quiet and reserved, perhaps introverted. I believe Scot would agree that we have a good father-son relationship. He knows he can ask me or tell me anything. He knows I love him and would do anything for him. Our relationship was forged during that year and a half of daily, close physical and emotional bonding. Even though the time and its challenges were demanding and uncertain, I credit it with fostering a relationship I wish I could have experienced growing up. Even here, as I close my eyes and think back on those days, I'm afraid I see them in a light that did not exist in real-time. How does one process the real-time valleys in such a way as to maintain a healthy mental approach to them?

After summer school, I had two semesters remaining. I felt like I could see the end of the tunnel. School went well. I did continue to succeed. I aced everything except one statistics course, where I pulled a B. I was OK with that. I realized from those final three semesters and summer school that I was no smarter than I had been in my two previous college stints- no smarter. By then, I was more motivated and driven. Whenever I thought about skipping a class, I saw myself burning a twenty-dollar bill. That was the actual monetary cost of every class session. This time I was paying for it all. I now had a motivation (a family including a son) that outweighed the fear of failure.

As the final semester began, I began thinking about life after Guilford. When I returned to Guilford the previous spring, I honestly thought about becoming a teacher. I wrote about that in my statement that accompanied my application for readmission. That didn't last long. My transcript shows no education courses, and I have no memory of ever being counseled or coached toward taking any education classes. Looking back from this distance, especially after working for over thirty years in that academic environment, I am surprised at that. I don't think I ever really had a desire to teach. When I was writing my application to get back in, it sounded good.

With only one semester left, I was a declared Sociology and Political Science double major. With only four months left in school, I realized I needed to look at job possibilities. I was way past ready to give up the newspaper route. Much like my earlier comments about going to college and getting out of the tobacco patches, I finally felt the same about the paper route and graduating from college. Two of my favorite professors at Guilford were Paul Zopf and Andy Gottschall. Paul was chair of the Sociology Department and a demographer with a Latin America specialty.

He was also the best-dressed and most organized teacher I ever had. After I went to work at the college, I would have opportunities to get to know both Paul and his wife, Evelyn, better. Andy was my academic advisor for most of my return to college. I am not sure how it came about. Andy would be the one who would open the door to my first professional job after Guilford.

Andy's father was one of the earliest participants in creating the National Conference of Christians and Jews, a non-profit organization dealing with social justice issues, particularly relating to faith-based matters and discrimination based on faith, race, and ethnicity. The NCCJ was headquartered in New York. It was founded in 1927 to counter a wave of anti-Catholicism and antisemitism in the United States. It has regional offices spread throughout the US. Andy followed in his father's footsteps and worked with NCCJ as a regional director before finding a home in the Sociology Dept. at Guilford. I do not recall the specifics. At some point during that final semester, Andy invited me to his office to talk about life after Guilford. It seems the Carolinas Regional Chapter of the NCCJ needed a director. The previous director had been promoted to the organization's Rocky Mountain Office in Denver. Andy thought I would be a good candidate for the job. How? Why? To this day, I have no idea. It was a surprise then, and it remains a mystery now. I knew nothing about the NCCJ. I only knew a little about the Jewish faith outside of what I had studied in Old Testament religion classes. I did not have a graduate degree. I was finishing a four-year BS that took me ten years to obtain. I was knocking it out of the park, grade-wise. Really? Was this one of those God-things? I don't know. If so, I have to consider it a precursor of things to come.

I never got the chance to ask Andy that question later when it finally occurred to me. I was too focused on getting a job to be concerned with the how and why. Andy passed away not long after graduation and during my time with NCCJ. Andy took me to Virginia to meet Dr. Peter Millette, a VP for NCCJ. Dr. Millette's' duties included supervising the director of the Carolinas Regional Office located in Greensboro and a separate office in Charlotte that worked just in Mecklenburg County as a United-Way agency. We met at the beautiful historic Roanoke Hotel in downtown Roanoke. Peter was there to manage a fund-raising dinner that evening.

Such subscription dinners were the primary fundraising tools for NCCJ chapters nationwide. Either the interview went well enough, or Peter was desperate and willing to rely on Andy's judgment. They offered me the job, and I took it. I would soon go to work in the office in downtown Greensboro as the NCCJ Carolinas Regional Director a week after graduation. I was on cloud nine. I had finally graduated from college- the first in my family to do so, even if it took me ten years to get a four-year degree. I had my first real professional job. I would soon go to work every day in a suit and a tie in the middle of the financial and business center of what was to me (still a poor kid from Goldsboro), a big city. I had a beautiful wife and a wonderful little boy, now two years old. Life was good all over. We still lived in a rented house. That, too, would change soon enough. And I was no longer getting up at 4:00 in the morning to deliver the Greensboro paper in all kinds of weather.

I will never forget my mother, sister, and brother-in-law from Goldsboro joining my little family and Becky's parents on the lawn at Guilford to watch me march onto the scene and cross the stage- a graduate of Guilford College. Paul Zopf was the commencement speaker. How appropriate. Like most commencement exercises, I remember nothing Paul said that morning. I remember the day and being so excited life was finally taking a turn in the right direction. Other than when Becky said "yes" seven years earlier, I had experienced a few moments that felt like that. And those precious moments of not just momentary exuberance but internalized high expectations always seemed to run afoul of reality. This time would be different. This time was more permanent- or was it?

TIME! It can be such a deceiving master. One has absolutely no control over it. It seems quite the contrary is true. When experiencing those times of trial, failure, and disappointment, it seems time stands still. Will this never end? Is "it" never going to get any better? I remember like it was yesterday, those feelings pervading my every waking thought during the period leading up to leaving my job at the bank and returning to college. Those days and weeks before moving back to Greensboro and starting classes were agonizing. They had the same sixty minutes and twenty-four hours all days have. But the emotional baggage carried into each day seemed like a ball and chain wrapped around the hands of the clock, not allowing time to move at its proper pace. Those valleys were too deep; the mountains that had to be crossed to escape were too steep.

Time does move on. Through whatever means that control time, or that time controls, the minutes and hours, days and weeks, after making the move to this next chapter in life, time picked up the pace. From the outset, the time spent with my son (except for those moments when we both were out-of-sorts) and the early successes in the classroom created a new daily perspective. Even the early morning regimen seemed more a minor nuisance than anything else. Even in the real-time of the day, I was keenly aware it was serving a meaningful purpose. I was good with that.

As time unfolded to encompass a year-and-a-half stint, it became evident that time was marching at a different pace. Those same minutes and hours, days and weeks, whose passage seemed to be thwarted by a ball and chain, now were flying by. I enjoyed being present to share my son's early awakening to life. I enjoyed the hours Becky and I had together. I was enjoying school- something I had not done in a long time-because I was succeeding. And it was all flying by. Those peaks and WOW experiences were exhilarating. In those moments, I was captivated by the exhilaration. I didn't notice TIME was deceiving me; that the terrain that stymied escaping from the depths of the valleys and prolonged that escape was the same landscape that can facilitate unexpected and dangerous slides back into the depths of the valley.

Yes! TIME can be a deceiving master. On one level, I understand the ebb and flow between peaks and valleys, between WOW moments and depths of despair. I struggle coming to terms with the deceitfulness of time within whose borders these emotions are manifested. Why must time be so unfair? Why can't it just allow life to unfold on a fair and even playing field? I don't know.

Chapter 15

COMING TO TERMS

THE JOY FROM the job offer from NCCJ and having a respectable job right out of college was short-lived. I soon found that most of my time would be spent fundraising to support a program that needed more program presence in the Triad. There was an active chapter in Charlotte. That was a separate entity, and that separation was made clear to me early on. Its primary source of financial support was the United Way, and its primary programming centered around social justice education aimed at high school students. I received little training or program support. My job was to get to know the right people in the Greensboro (not Triad) business community to be able to mobilize them when the time came to put on the annual NCCJ Brotherhood Dinner- a $50 a plate dinner "honoring" a highly visible public citizen. With the help of my boss in Richmond, we recruited a well-known and respected businessperson to chair the event. They would use their name and connections to help bring in the higher rollers. Their success would enable us to fill the room with others who believed in the cause and wanted to be seen associating with that group of leaders. It was a tried-and-true fundraising program used by NCCJ and many other NPOs nationwide.

My nature as an introvert and having no experience working with or associating with this spectrum of the socio-economic class made it difficult for me to be successful in that enterprise. That, coupled with the sociologist in me, was the perfect brew for a failed experience. My immediate supervisor, Dr. Millette, would come down occasionally, once or twice a year. He would be here for the actual dinner events. Between visits to Greensboro, I would meet him at the Hotel Roanoke when he worked on that dinner preparation.

Midway through my two years with NCCJ, I asked for and received permission to move the office from its downtown Greensboro location, where it had been for many years. We needed help making a budget, and rent in the historic Southeastern Building was going up. I found a smaller office space in a one-floor building across the main entrance from Guilford College. By this time, Becky and I had bought a brand-new house near Kernersville and moved out of the rental house. The new NCCJ location cut nearly fifteen minutes off my commute. It also placed the office sufficiently distanced from downtown Greensboro that one could legitimately think it was a Triad office. If we were the Carolinas Regional Office for NCCJ, we ought to have some semblance of a regional presence. I was now conducting a small reading program featuring NCCJ literature around the "brotherhood" theme. We were getting into schools in the Triad area and Durham and Goldsboro-cities where I had some personal connections. We produced a brief tv PR campaign around the theme using the Wee Pals cartoon characters. The folks at WXII-TV in Winston-Salem did that for us. We wanted to create a real regional presence with some substantive programming. I was convinced that I could help open fundraising doors.

Well, it was all a total bust. Although I had been permitted to move the office, there needed to be more support for focusing on regional program development before fundraising. I understood the budgetary implications of a program-first approach. I understood it meant asking National to underwrite some of the costs in the near term. I lost that battle and, with it, any desire to continue. I will always remember meeting with Dr. Millette and him telling me it looked like they (he and NCCJ) had made a mistake in my hiring. I was grossly hurt and offended at the time. In retrospect, he was right. I was in way over my head at the outset. I am forever grateful to Andy Gotschall and Dr. Millette for giving me that chance. They should have known better. They took a chance, and it didn't work. [I would be remiss if I did not acknowledge NCCJ has had a successful presence in Greensboro for many years since those days. It did move back to near downtown Greensboro and now is the Piedmont Triad NCCJ Chapter.

Once again, what looked like a bright and shining future had imploded. Once again, I failed to capitalize on an opportunity placed before me. I was even stupid enough to quit the job before I had another job. That may be a moot point. I suspect Dr. Rhodes would have fired me soon enough. I left mid-March 1979, just a few weeks after that year's Brotherhood Citation Dinner in February. I got a manual labor job working at a metal fabrication plant, assembling metal ashtrays and airplane seat hinges. (Yes- in those days, you could smoke on board the plane.) It was hard work. I came home daily with numerous small, razor-sharp cuts on my hands from the sharp edges of the pieces I was assembling. I got up every morning, dreading every minute of the day ahead. Once again, though, Becky was a rock. She never questioned what I did. She understood how I got to that point. She continued to go to her job at the hospital.

Looking back, I am stunned at how stupid I continued to be. When I resigned from NCCJ, Becky was six months pregnant with Courtney, our second child. We had bought a house just a few months earlier. Now I was quitting a job with nothing to go to, with a mortgage and second child on the way. I don't know what possessed me. That was not the first time. It would not be the last. What I believed to be a well-deserved peak in life was soon followed by days and weeks of valleys, followed by another scrape with the bottom. I could write a whole epistle about the circumstances and rationale surrounding these decisions and what I did or did not learn from them. That's for another day-perhaps. Still, in retrospect, time seemed to pick and choose its pace.

Maybe something would turn up. I submitted applications. I got no interviews. Finally, after about a month at the fabricating plant, I decided to deliver a resume to Guilford College. I didn't know if they had anything I might be qualified for. You know the story by now. I was in and out of Guilford three times over ten years and did so poorly that even acing all but one course in my final four semesters left me graduating with barely a 2.12 GPA. I often thought I might like to finish my career at Guilford. I had no idea what the rest of my career might look like; Maybe there would be a way to get back to Guilford to close out my working life and say "thank you" for giving me those opportunities. So, I walked in and dropped off a resume with the receptionist in New Garden Hall, the main administration building. I had no idea who to see, so I just asked the receptionist if she could see that it found its way to whoever was the appropriate person. What followed could never have been imagined.

Within a week, I received a call from the college. I cannot remember who called. They wanted me to come in and complete a formal application if I was interested in applying for the Director of Financial Aid position. I had plenty of experience in dealing with Financial Aid directors. I had yet to learn exactly what they did all day. But it was Guilford. It was a real job. And I was motivated. I completed the application and went home to wait.

The Farlex Dictionary of Idioms defines "coming to terms" as the act of "beginning or making an effort to understand, accept, and deal with a difficult or problematic person, thing, or situation." The American Heritage Dictionary of Idioms says it means to "reconcile oneself to, as in 'He'd been trying to come to terms with his early life'."

When beginning this exercise, I had some idea of the story that awaited my exposing it. I had a good notion of the factual content that warranted commitment to the manuscript. As it unfolded and re-unfolded, I saw a reasonable chronological telling of the story. When the first telling was drafted, I thought I had a workable timeframe for each chapter and a list of descriptive chapter headings.

"Coming to Terms" turned out to be one of the shorter chapters in textual content. I've often heard (and I am pretty sure the reader has heard) the expression, "don't judge a book by its cover." My adaptation of that advice would be, "don't

judge a book (or chapter) by the number of words contained therein." Reliving the years leading up to the two-year window covered in this chapter brought about a seemingly never-ending series of mental calisthenics. One WOW moment was constantly followed, eventually, by a time of utter disappointment or embarrassment. A rolling tide of failure or disappointing behavior soon washed away one uplifting peak experience. The emotional impact from one never seemed to last as long or carry the same motivating drive as the debilitating after-effects of the other. Oops- there it is again- 'never seemed to last as long.' Time- playing its ugly game again. One set of feel-good experiential inputs fading away much faster than the journey up from the valley that always returns to recapture the scene.

So, in early May 1979, I was perched and ready to take a huge step forward in my professional life and everything that degree could provide in my personal and family life. I had weathered the severing of the cord with NCCJ. I had acknowledged both the Conference and I had probably made a mistake. The Conference would move on and be fine. I was ready to move on. I was waiting for the college to give me that opportunity, and it looked like just a paperwork formality. I had "come to terms" with my situation. I believed all I needed was for Guilford College to give me a chance to prove it.

I had no idea that "coming to terms" would be a much more open-ended process, with which time would continue to wreak havoc. Forty-four years later, I am still "coming to terms." I now wonder if time will win out one way or another.

Chapter 16

MAYBE THERE'S A MISSION HERE

SPOILER ALERT!!!! Up to now, I have attempted to recount stories and recall issues in chronological order. The chapters of this effort have correctly reflected the years of my early life. From now on, the chapters may be less cohesively structured. The next two chapters and the first part of Chapter 18 cover my 30 ½ years on staff at Guilford College. There is a logical break that results in the next two chapters. However, beyond that, I have made no serious effort to be meticulous about the proper sequencing of the stories. Some logical sequencing will occur simply because it has been easy to remember things in that order. In many cases, I don't recall exactly when this or that happened, just that it did occur within the general timeframe being recounted. I hope this lack of sequential accuracy does not get in the way of telling what I think is essential.

I was thrilled when Guilford hired me as its Director of Financial Aid. I needed a real job. But it was more than that. I was going to work at Guilford College- where I had failed twice before succeeding on the road to graduation. Until now, my road to success had been more detours and potholes than four-lane direct routes. I was on the verge of a new and exciting path. I didn't know much about the actual job ahead. But it was my alma mater. I wasn't going to get rich. I was OK with that. For the first time, I felt like I was carrying my fair share of the financial load in our household. For the first time since my first departure from Guilford, I felt like I could be proud of my station in life when I reflected on it in comparison with my high school friends. NOTE: <u>This has always been a significant problem- a lifetime of comparing my life, my situation, and my status to that of schoolmates about whom I knew very little, other than the obvious public persona they presented. I have spent a lifetime living in that mistaken view of life and the world.</u>

I reported to work on May 1, 1979. The Financial Aid Office (FAO) was just me and a secretary/receptionist/right-hand assistant, Dianne Harrison. Ms. Harrison, or "Di" as she liked to be called, had worked at Guilford for several years, starting at the downtown campus in the Registrar's Office. There had been a steady turnover in the FAO for a few years before my arrival. That May's graduation was one week after my arrival. For those graduating seniors, I was the fourth FA Director they had seen in their four years at "Guilco." Over the years, as my tenure there grew, I may have accomplished little else in managing the financial aid operation at the college, but I certainly rectified the steady turnover trend.

Unlike today, much of the work in assessing students' eligibility for financial aid and packaging and managing post-awards paperwork was just that- paperwork. Today, nearly everything is digital. Back then, it was all paper. I was a good learner and a quick study. It didn't take long for me to feel comfortable in my surroundings and my responsibilities. However, it was a daunting challenge. We were understaffed as the college began to grow its adult student population and the federal student loan programs ratcheted up. I didn't mind, though. I was doing an important job, and I "felt like somebody."

I'll never forget the night my boss stopped by my door. It was probably 6:30 or 7:00. I was still at my desk, hoping to get out before too long. This was not unusual. It wasn't until years later that I realized how I had taken my wife for granted in those years and how I had failed my kids regularly by not being home during those precious hours. At some point, I realized my mistake. It was water under the bridge by then. As much as I loved my time at Guilford and appreciate what the college did for me and my family, I regret I allowed myself to fall into that pit so early in my time there. My boss stopped by to ask a question. He had seen the lights on in my office. He popped in the door and asked me if I ever watched the Olympics. I wondered where he was going with this, but I said, "yes." I am a big sports fan and watch all kinds of sports. He then asked me if I had ever seen a runner compete in the 100-meter dash and the marathon. Of course, I said "no,"- to which he responded, "and neither can you." He was an early arriver in the mornings. He observed that most mornings, my car was one of only a handful already in the staff parking lot when he arrived. He also noted that this evening, like many others, I was one of the few staff still in their offices. He reminded me that I, too, could not run both the dash and the marathon. I needed to decide if I was in this thing for the near term or the long haul. I understood what he was telling me. It took me 12-15 years on the job to internalize it to the point of moderating my behavior accordingly. I regret I was so slow on the uptake. On later occasions, when he and I would have conversations, I would explain to him I was only doing what I had to do to get the job done. He told me, "sometimes you have to let it break before those

in positions of authority will listen and respond appropriately."
Fortunately, about midway through my 30 years on the job, I
began to understand the advice. As the role of the FAO grew
within developing enrollment management and student financial services umbrellas, and as the student population grew to
double the size when I first went to work, we raised the staffing
to nearly what was sufficient.

My boss was not only a wonderful boss but a great mentor
as well. We met years before I went to work at the college. He
was my German professor for two semesters during my first
year. I enjoyed his classes, but I was not a good student. He was
not particularly good at heeding his own advice, though. He
had his baggage to carry. A few years after my reporting chain
had been altered and I was reporting to Jim Newlin, the college CFO, I learned, while traveling on a recruiting trip, that
my former boss had committed suicide. He dealt with chronic
depression for many years. I did not know that at the time. I
was stunned when I got the news. While that experience was
not my first encounter with the suicide of someone I knew, it
was the first time a dear friend, mentor, and colleague had taken
that path. I had not seen it coming. It scared me. The fact that
it scared me more than grieved me still gives me pause.

The years at Guilford moved along at a brisk pace. As I
look back, sometimes it felt like the days (some days) would
never end. Then, suddenly, where did the time go? How did the
years get past me so quickly? (There's that phantom again-time-
always present, but rarely conspicuous). It serves no purpose
here to get too bogged down in the day-to-day minutia of the
job. I went to work. I did well what the college had hired me to
do. I kept my head below the firing line when it came to campus
politics, a word to the wise my former Poli Sci professor gave

me before I accepted the job. There would come a time after I had been on the job for a sufficient period that such avoidance of the intra-squabbling was hard to maintain. I tried my best. That may be why I could keep my job for 30 years- never advancing far in the administration. Nevertheless, those years were filled with good and bad memories, some of which are worth reporting herein as they relate to the over-arching question at hand.

Those early years were full of change, new experiences, peaks, and valleys at home and work. That period from quitting my job at the Conference and going to work at Guilford was full of intended and unintended changes and consequences. No one in their right mind would leave a job while expecting a second child in a few short months. I cannot, for the life of me, understand how Becky did not cut her losses then and there. But she didn't. Fortunately, the opportunity at Guilford did materialize, and it looked like we might get through that time unscathed. Six weeks after starting the new gig at Guilford, we moved into our new house and welcomed our daughter, Courtney, into our family. I'll always remember the race one night from our little house just outside Kernersville to Wesley Long Hospital in Greensboro. Our Toyota station wagon didn't stop at even one stop sign or traffic light on its way. Becky, like her mom, was designed to make babies. She was well on her way to welcoming Courtney when we arrived at the hospital. She went straight from the ER to Labor & Delivery and the delivery room- no pit stops anywhere. By the time I could change into my scrubs, we were becoming a family of four.

Courtney's arrival was a welcome sight for many reasons; Becky had significant health issues throughout the pregnancy. She was diagnosed with Meniere's Disease, a serious inner ear imbalance (vertigo) situation. It was unusual for a young woman to encounter this illness. Its typical debilitating effects and routine body changes experienced during pregnancy made it difficult for Becky for several months. She was confined to bed (and a darkened room) on multiple occasions during that period. Sometime after the delivery, Becky would have surgery to implant a stint in the inner ear to reduce fluid accumulation. Over the years, she has occasionally had minor reoccurrences of the dizziness associated with the syndrome, but nothing like during her pregnancy.

While Courtney's addition to the family was a joyous time, beneath the glow and warmth of her arrival, I again began to hear the demons calling. In my quiet moments late at night or during the day when something went askew, I asked myself, "What the hell am I doing? I had no idea how to be a good father to this child. I was already wrestling with my shortcomings in fathering my son. What did I know about being a dad to this beautiful little creature? One of the reasons I fell into such a work-focused routine was that fear. If I could be absorbed in my work, I didn't have to worry about my shortcomings at home. I'm afraid I may have allowed that diversion to take root and govern way too much of my work and family life over the next twenty years.

This was all happening while I was discovering one thing after another that was not right with our new house. We had floor molding that needed to be installed correctly. We had a water well that was running out of water after just a few months, or the pump was not functioning correctly. I was at a loss for dealing with those kinds of issues. I could not get anywhere with the realtor who sold us the house or the contractor. This was a world I knew nothing about, and, as usual, I was not good at asking for help. So, we were in a new house less than a few months, with two small children, financial issues mounting due to house and health issues, a desire to get the job done well in my new career, and a sense that a distance between me and Becky was beginning to surface- something I had not felt before. I do not mean to imply that this feeling suggested I was beginning to feel less in love with my bride. No! I began to feel my incompetence had caused this crescendo of causes and effects. She deserved better. Our children deserved better. I was dangerously afraid Becky would come to this same conclusion, and I would have no choice- she would make that choice for us.

We continued to function in this fog for a couple of years. I have no clue how we survived emotionally, other than Becky, as I have said before, was a Rock. Even though she had her issues to deal with, she never struck out at me or hinted our lives together might end. After two or three years, we moved back to Greensboro to be closer to both jobs. Rather than trying to sell the house, we rented it to the family who lived next door. Their lease was ending, and they were going to have to move. It seemed like a great plan. The renters would pay our mortgage payments, and we would rent a house in Greensboro. I had worked out a deal with a fellow staffer at the college to rent a house he owned. Later we would move into a college-owned house right across the street from the college.

As has often been the story of my life, I placed too much faith in someone else doing the right thing and did not face the music head-on at the outset. Within a few months of moving, our renters began missing rent payments. We had always been on a thin financial margin. We had no room to make both mortgage and rent payments. In short order, we were in default on our mortgage, and the house was being repossessed. Ultimately, the neighbors who had moved into our house were evicted, and the bank sold the house at auction. Fortunately, it sold for enough to pay off our loan, and we were clear of that obligation.

So, we were back in Greensboro. We both liked our jobs. But, because of a chain of financial circumstances and bad choices associated with them, we were still not in a good place- I was not in a good place.

In these early years, with just me and Di in the office, I was responsible for all financial aid awarding. Dianne took a lot of phone calls and walk-in student and parent traffic. She was a Godsend. As the years went by and the size of the staff grew, well into the latter half of my time there, I would become less involved in day-to-day student contact and more of a policy and personnel manager. Over the years, Di went back to college (while working her full-time job) and was promoted to Director of Financial Aid as my responsibilities and title changed to Associate Dean of Enrollment and then to Director of Student Financial Services. I missed those earlier times. Still today, I stay in touch with several students from the 80s and 90s.

Three years after joining the staff at Guilford, Becky and I celebrated our 10th wedding anniversary. That was important for us. We looked around and noticed how few of our cohort group had survived marriage to their 10th anniversary. So, we saved a little, financed a little, and took what, for us at that time, was a big celebratory vacation. We took a 7-day cruise to the Bahamas. That may seem insignificant nowadays. Becky grew up in a solid middle-class North Carolina farm family. She didn't go without anything of importance.

On the other hand, she had traveled little other than to places where her dad was competing with fox hounds. My travel had been limited to my summer Encampment experience in high school, the NYC trip my first year at Guilford, and a handful of college admission recruiting drives to northern Virginia after I joined the staff at Guilford. A 7-day cruise to the Bahamas was something neither of us could have ever imagined a few short years earlier. Becky's parents were gracious to babysit for us. The reason I single out this occasion is simple. I had never seen Becky so beautiful in all the years I had known her. I had never seen anything so beautiful. Perhaps because we both were so busy with work and trying to be good parents to two small children, I just had not stopped long enough to really see the woman God had blessed me with. Don't get me wrong. I knew she was beautiful. After all, when I was 21 years old and watched her walk down the hall in the Whitaker Center for the first time, I knew she was beautiful.

I didn't know then just how deep that beauty dwelt and how unassuming she was about it all. Those seven days, with all the physical communion with one another and the emotional bonding that manifested itself, took my love and appreciation for my wife to a new level. Still today, sometimes, I catch myself closing my eyes and seeing Becky at the top of the gangplank as we embarked on our adventure. Parts of me still respond in ways they haven't reacted in years. Other parts of me simply tingle in a way I cannot adequately describe. You would understand if you had seen her then and know her today. We are 50 years older now; she is still the most beautiful woman I have ever seen- the force that keeps me girding up for the struggle.

That's one of the peaks – knowing every day I get to share time and space with the most amazing creation (in all its man-ifestations), God has ever brought into my life. Where is the valley? At the outset, I raised the question of peaks and valleys. One of the recurring valleys is the nagging question- how did

I come to be so fortunate, and why (and how) have I so often failed to be so worthy? How often has Becky had to bear the brunt of my failures? I reflect on the hopes and dreams that were so much a part of our lives in those days. Forty years later, I wither in that reflection- recounting all the missed opportunities, the failed attempts, the unattempted openings. She deserved so much better. Yet, she has never beaten me up over any of this. I hate, I absolutely hate, that I have not been able to give her more of the worldly things we "dreamed" about in those years- more cruises with her standing at the top of the gangplank looking just like that image of perfection. She insists it's OK. She tells me she could not be happier with her circumstances in life. Her actions mesh with her words. She has never given me any reason to believe otherwise.

One of the perks I would enjoy in my new job at Guilford was occasional business travel to state, regional, or national conferences. Contrary to what many think, these were business engagements, and honest work was done. There could also be terrific opportunities to socialize with friends and colleagues and see some sights. Socializing is not one of my favorite things to do. I can maneuver as necessary in such venues. It is not my preference. I discovered that, on occasion, when the destination and the calendar presented themselves, I could arrange for nice short-term family vacations around my business trip. I could arrange the travel and lodging so it would cost the college no more than it would cost me alone. Instead of staying in the high-dollar conference hotels, my family and I could stay in a Days Inn or similar lodging for no more (often less) than my room at the conference center. Often, we would drive the family minivan and cost the college no more for mileage than airfare for me alone would be. Throughout our children's growing up years, we could take them to places we would not otherwise have visited as a family. Becky would do the tourist thing with the kids while I was in meetings. I made it clear to my family and my boss I was not skipping important conference events to do this. (I know some colleagues did, in fact, skip sessions regularly to go on purely pleasure romps with other colleagues). I would join the family for evening outings, and we would extend the trips a few days, on our budget, when the city's offerings warranted such extensions. We shared experiences in D.C., Philadelphia, Dallas, Atlanta, Miami, Denver, St. Louis, and Los Angeles. Sometimes it would just be Becky and me. Becky joined me on one such trip to Hawaii.

One such occasion the family did not join me on was a 15-day trip to the then U.S.S.R. with a busload of college educators and administrators from around the country. This was the summer of 1986, just a few weeks after the Chernobyl nuclear accident in April. Stanley Frank, a wealthy Greensboro businessman and long-time trustee at the college, had endowed a scholarship and mentoring program for entrepreneurially minded students with a passion for capitalism and free enterprise. Since I ran the financial aid program at the college, and since the college couldn't decide just how to structure the program, it fell on my desk for a couple of years until we could arrange for an academic department to take charge. Not long after assuming responsibility for the program, a flyer came across my desk about this trip. It came out of the blue. My first impulse was to toss it. I didn't. I thought, if I am going to run this program about scholarship and entrepreneurship, wouldn't it be informative for me to witness, up close and personal, the antithesis of American capitalism- Soviet communism? We had no budget for such a thing. This was one of those rare occasions where I did not hesitate to ask for help. I took the brochure to my boss and pled my case. She told me to write the request with adequate cause and documentation. She would see what she could do. The rest is history.

Colleges were more financially stable then, and she could be persuasive. (I think she pitched it as a way to reward me for work beyond what I was getting paid as much as anything directly related to the program.) At any rate, I spent fifteen days riding buses, planes, and trains with colleagues from colleges and universities around the country, seeing a good portion of western Russia. We visited Moscow, Rostov-on-Don, Sochi, and Leningrad (now St. Petersburg). The trip was rerouted days before our departure to Moscow because of the Chernobyl nuclear disaster. We were scheduled to have visits downwind from the nuclear site. There is not enough time or space herein to go into the trip's details.

Aside from the particulars that did relate to my rationale for going, I came home with one substantial life-altering reckoning. When I landed in New York on my way home from Moscow, I had the visual image of seeing the Pope. When he arrived at places he was visiting in his official duties as Pope, he would kneel and kiss the pavement at the bottom of the steps. That's what I felt like doing when I stepped on the ground in New York. My college experience broadened my horizons. Nothing had prepared this kid from The Project for what he had experienced in Russia. I felt like kissing the ground. Becky and I had often talked about wanting our children to have travel opportunities we had never had. Some of that we were covering with my professional travel opportunities. This experience changed my thinking. This kind of international exposure was no longer an optional offering in their growing up. No- it became necessary-and not just a 10-day sightseeing group trip with thirty other vacationing teenagers. No, they needed to experience life in a strange place, a different culture. They needed to experience that the world does not revolve around them and their homeland. They needed to experience being more than a five-minute drive to the nearest McDonalds. Becky and I agreed we would do whatever we could to open doors for this to happen. We still believe it was a good decision.

Scot was a bright kid and rather tall for his age. We found he was having a tough time at school in that, to use a cliché, he walked to the beat of a different drummer. By the time he reached the 4th grade, we were wrestling with how to address the fact his day-to-day school situation was not speaking to his needs. So, we began looking at private school options. There were several in the Greensboro area. We applied to a couple, and it looked like we would send him to a highly regarded private school on the north side of Greensboro. Just a few days before school started, I was conversing with an accounting professor at the college and a man of faith in whom I had considerable confidence. I was explaining our dilemma. He listened attentively and then made a suggestion. We were both in the business of helping young adults make good decisions about their higher education experience- him from an academic program standpoint and me from a cost/investment standpoint. He told me that, in his opinion, the choices we make as parents at that developmental time in our children's lives are far more important than the decision as to where they might go to college six to ten years later. Somehow, that resonated with me. His children were attending Wesleyan Christian Academy in High Point. WCA is a well-respected faith-based school.

We had applied there, and Scot had been accepted. Fortunately, at that late hour, we were able to activate his acceptance, and he enrolled there just a couple of days later. Courtney would follow him there a few years later. That decision had significant financial implications, implications not easily accepted given what I have already mentioned. Driving older cars, resoling shoes multiple times, and rarely eating out became the norm for us. Becky and I were convinced it was the right thing to do. By this time, we were consciously working to grow our focus on our faith walk. As the next few years unfolded, that decision to involve our family with the Wesleyan community proved to be a vital step in a particularly good direction. It was the right decision. I am forever grateful to my friend for pointing to that door.

A couple of years after this transfer to Wesleyan, when Scot was twelve years old, we began to explore the notion of his going abroad for his sixteenth birthday. The thought was he could pick the place, and I would arrange a host family for a six-week stay. If we could arrange it so, the host family would have a corresponding teenager who would accompany Scot home after his six weeks. This teenager would stay with us for six weeks, and we would make every effort to expose him to a variety of American life. Scot had to choose and let me know by the summer of his fourteenth birthday. I could use my Guilford connections to track down a suitable link. One of the many blessings of my time at Guilford was the international exposure. We had many students from various parts of the world. The Quakers, although their numbers were small, were well connected globally. As it turned out, Scot wanted to go to Paris.

I was able to connect him with a family from a small suburb of Paris. A Guilford's IT department member had a sister who was married to a Frenchman. They had children, one of whom was a teenage son the same age as Scot. Scot lived with the family for six weeks. Arnaud, the French teenager, came to Kernersville and lived with us for six weeks. That part of the experience could have been less awkward. Arnaud and Scot were different, with wildly divergent interests. By then, we were living in the farmhouse, and it was still a big mess. Given our decision regarding our kids' education, we made a few cosmetic renovations to the old farmhouse. It was still a mess in many ways. I was embarrassed. I know Scot had to be, but he never said a word. I have never moved past that summer and the embarrassment I felt for myself and my family.

While at Guilford, I occasionally ran into high school friends from Goldsboro. One of the more memorable such occasions involved Edie Hampshire. You may remember I mentioned her earlier in this epistle. I was sitting in my office one day, and the phone rang. The receptionist downstairs was calling regarding a guest in the lobby. The Financial Aid Office shared space in the New Garden Hall administration building with Admission and other functions. The receptionist wanted to know if my name was Gene Gurley or if I might be related to Gene Gurley. The placard on the wall at her desk listing all the staff had my name: Anthony Gurley. A woman in the lobby from Alaska with her daughter was waiting for their Admission appointment. The lady had inquired about Anthony Gurley, the Director of Financial Aid. She told the receptionist she had gone to high school with Gene Gurley and wondered if Anthony might be Gene. She seemed to remember Gene had attended Guilford College. I was thrilled. I knew exactly who was in the lobby. Of course, Gene and Anthony were the same person. My full name is Anthony Eugene Gurley. I grew up

Gene and always wanted to be called Anthony. It was when I went to work at North Carolina National Bank (NCNB) that I could pull off the switch. I had the bank put Anthony E. Gurley on my desk name plate. Since then, I have been Anthony to everyone other than my immediate family and high school friends. To them, I still answer as Gene.

I rushed down the stairs and greeted an old friend. Edie's husband had been in the Air Force and then worked as a civilian contractor for the DOD. They lived in Alaska for many years, where Edie taught elementary school. Edie was on campus with one of her daughters, looking at Guilford. That daughter did attend and graduate from my alma mater. I cannot tell you how happy seeing Edie that day made me, and later, to see her daughter now and then on campus. Edie was still that beautiful, engaging girl I first met in the fourth grade and continued to admire all through high school. This, my friends, was one of those "peaks." Edie and I have stayed in touch since those days, as our high school class has enjoyed class reunions.

I have gone off on a tangent and gotten ahead of myself. That may be because I am approaching a period I prefer to skip over. I must include this part of the story in the interest of full disclosure. I have noted my instinct for introversion and shyness. Those personality traits have always been a part of me. A curious thing happens more frequently than I can understand, and it did so early in my career in financial aid at Guilford. As the Director of FA, I established membership in state, regional, and national professional associations. As noted earlier, I would attend annual conferences and workshops and participate in association work, particularly at the state and regional levels.

Early in my work at Guilford, I became involved professionally in our state association. I was elected to serve as an officer in that association just a few years after entering the profession. I did not seek the job. In retrospect, given how poor a manager I was in my own household, I should have declined to have my name placed on the ballot. I didn't. I was elected. I see nothing to be gained by going into the details of what transpired over the next several months relative to my function in that role. Before the year was out, I resigned from my position in the association. I was an improper choice for that position. My poor behavior and performance in that trusted role warranted my removal from office. The association board would have removed me from office if I had not resigned. Let me be clear. I did not lose my job at Guilford. I was never reprimanded or punished in any way. In thirty years of annual financial audits, occasional program reviews, and annual staff evaluations, there was **never** any inkling of any professional misconduct associated with my duties at the college.

This experience, for which I accept total responsibility, changed my life. A life already dogged by a sense of failure and underperformance now added to the mix a loss of trust and respect- personally and among friends and colleagues I admired and respected. My professional career suddenly had no upper mobility. I loved my years at Guilford and had no desire to go elsewhere. I missed the professional interaction and development that disappeared afterward. I attended association conferences and workshops as needed but always felt like an outsider, almost like a pariah. I had let my colleagues down. I never outlived that feeling. I still wonder how my professional life might have been different had I not made that series of bad choices. No one can ever know how these things affect the course of life. I don't know what experiences I avoided that were even more detrimental to my professional or personal health. What I do know is that, once again, I was embarrassed and ashamed. Once again, I failed to take advantage of an opportunity to raise my position. Once again, I failed. That memory has haunted me every day since.

One redeeming quality in all this, during these early years and extending throughout my time at Guilford, was the privilege of meeting and developing long-lasting relationships with some wonderful young people and, in some cases, young adults. When I find myself in one of those valley times, I try to return to the memories of my engagement with these folks and relive those good times.

I am reminded of the Big Mouth Frog that sat on my desk for many years. My daughter "bequeathed" it to me when she went off to college (a little bit after the period covered in this chapter; still relevant.) The frog was a green ceramic creature about the size of my fist with a big open mouth. I have no idea where it came from. Courtney used it as a soap dish in her bathroom. When she left for college, she gave it to me. I told her I would use it as a paperclip holder on my desk at the college, and that I did. It morphed into something far more significant than a paperclip holder after I added it to my desktop. It became a daily reminder for me of what my real calling at the college was.

I was paid to see that all financial aid matters were executed correctly. I did that. My real job, though, was kissing Big Mouth Frogs. By that, I mean listening to, embracing, and encouraging every single student who showed up at my desk. Their visits to my office often started with some financial aid question or paperwork matter. However, as often as not, the conversations moved on to other matters equally, usually more important. We would talk about all kinds of things that were on their minds. I learned early on not to judge. I rarely even offered any profound solutions. What I did was listen. I made sure they knew I understood. I often shared my story about taking ten years to get a four-year degree. I made sure they knew my door was always open. I learned I could not predict who would do or be what. I could not separate the wheat from the chaff. But I could kiss every big mouth frog that sat down at my desk, knowing everyone had the potential to turn into an amazing prince or princess one day. Even now, as I try to capture some of this history and help me weigh the decisions before me, I think of these memories and those frogs.

Allow me to share a few memories.

Several years after I retired from college, I received a call from one of those students. Micah Rushing wanted to meet for breakfast sometime. He just wanted to chat. Micah had a challenging time at Guilford. A stud athlete, he was dismissed from the college for reasons not important to this writing. When he met the college's requirements to allow him to return, he still had the matter of how to pay for it. I had forgotten about some of that story. Micah had not. He wanted to remind me of that time in his life and say, "Thank you." He reminded me of our meeting when he was trying to prepare to return to Guilco. He had no money. His mother couldn't help him to any great extent. She knew he wanted to finish what he had started but feared it was impossible. As Micah recounted the story, we met in my office and talked at some length. By the end of the meeting, I assured Micah that finances would not stand in the way of his return to Guilford. We could work it out. We still needed to figure out all the details but we could work it out. Micah left my office relieved.

What I didn't know then, and what Micah wanted to tell me that morning over breakfast, was what happened when he left my office. He went to his car in the parking lot outside my office and called his mother. He told her he had just left the financial aid director's office, and everything would be OK. He was going to be able to come back to Guilford. Scholarships, student loans, and some campus work would make it happen. Micah told me his mother cried over the phone. When he told me this story, I cried over breakfast. Micah and I have stayed in touch over the years since, mainly through Facebook.

Micha has gone on to pursue an interest (and talent) he had during that time- having little or nothing to do with his specific academic program at Guilford. Micah has developed quite a following as a barber. But not just one who cuts hair. No, Micah is an artist. He has traveled the world, working with numerous well-known celebs. His "Undefeated" brand has captured the imagination. Through all this, he has not abandoned his responsibility as a loving father. As he has grown personally and professionally, he is instilling in his daughter those values that helped him get through that difficult time in his life. I am so immensely proud of Micah.

A little over a year ago, Becky and I attended a fundraising dinner and celebration hosted by Dr. Beatrice Juncadella. Dr. Bea, or just Bea as I call her, is an accomplished pediatrician here in the Triad. I first met Bea when she was applying to Guilford College. Bea and her family managed to leave Nicaragua when she was in high school during the civil war unrest in the 1980s. Her parents were accomplished professionals and realized there was no future for them and their children in the midst of the violence in their country. They came to North Carolina and started a new life, being welcomed into a faith community in the Charlotte area. Bea did enroll at Guilford. She was not only very bright and an astute student, she was also a talented volleyball player. Because of the nature of the paperwork and never-ending issues associated with the financial aid process and the cost of a private college experience, Bea and I would see each other often. I was fascinated by her story, and she was grateful for my understanding and willingness to do what I could to assist her through the maze. Before too long, we were becoming friends. She met my family, and that friendship extended to both families.

I will never forget the day Bea came into my office in tears. She had left a class with a religion professor and didn't know what to do. Bea was/is a mighty woman of God. She lives out her faith every day. She did then. Her problem, as she explained it, her problem then was that the professor was telling her things she should believe that were inconsistent with what she did believe. And she was in no way inclined to change her beliefs. By this time, she had decided to be a doctor, a pediatrician. She could not perform poorly in class. She needed the highest grades to get into medical school. We talked a bit and then prayed together, something that did not often happen with students in the financial aid office. Some weeks later, Bea stopped by the office again. Her mood was much more upbeat (more like the Bea I have grown to know over the years). I asked her if she had figured out how to solve her problem. She had. She told me she would tell the professor what he wanted to hear and then go about believing what she knew in her heart to be right. She not only got an A in that course, she also graduated with a stellar academic career from the Brody School of Medicine at East Carolina University.

Dr. Bea never gave up her dream of being a medical missionary in Nicaragua. Beginning with a first mission trip with a couple of friends and a few hundred dollars many years ago, she has built a free-standing staffed clinic, a church, a scholarship program for students to go to university in Managua, and a soccer league. She takes teams of dozens of volunteers to the village several times each year. They conduct bible schools and help build and rehab houses. Bea blessed me by allowing me to assist in preparing her first 501c3 paperwork to secure official IRS recognition as a charitable medical ministry. She and her whole family have led this effort and built a safe place to administer much-needed medical care and, more importantly, be the hands and feet of God in the regions so in need of that Presence. I am so grateful for Bea's influence in my life. She has been a ray of hope and inspiration. I pray that God will continue to bless her and her work richly.

Just last week, I was on the phone with another former student with whom I have stayed in touch since his graduation in 1989. Chris was one of those rarities- an African American student from West Virginia. For a time, Guilford had a strong recruiting pipeline for top WV scholars. Chris was one of those. Chris is a striking presence, physically. When he walked into a room, everyone noticed. He didn't play football, but you would swear he was a stud linebacker. And he had the smile of a Cheshire cat. From his initial appearance, he had me. I met a few students who made the kind of lasting impression on me that Chris did. So much so when I decided to create Motivation Ministries in 2008, several years after he graduated from Guilford, Chris was the first person I asked to join my Board of Directors. I remember going home from work one day, some years after Chris was well on his way in his career and my daughter was in her teenage years. I don't remember what triggered the thought, but I told Becky I had experienced one of those epiphanic moments. I told her if our daughter came home one day with a "Chris" and told us this is who she was going to spend her life with, I would have no qualms. I could think of many young Caucasian men that I would dread the thought of her introducing to us as her husband-to-be. I don't know the significance of that realization, but it has surfaced occasionally over the years. Chris and I stay in touch. I count him as a dear friend. He was the most helpful member of my board during the Motivation years. I regret I could not produce at the level Chris had bought into. He has shown himself to be highly successful as a business coach. I was not one of his success stories.

Indulge me by allowing one more trip down memory lane.

I met Ron Davidson when he enrolled at Guilford through the Center for Continuing Education (CCE), our adult enrollment program. Ron had returned from the Army and decided to go to college. He wasn't sure what he wanted to do, but college seemed like the best route to get there. Like the other stories herein, we met when Ron showed up in my office with questions about some of the financial aid paperwork. Right off the bat, I like him. I liked his story and how he was changing the direction of some of that story. Ron was intelligent and hardworking. He also seemed a bit shy and reserved. I could relate.

We would see other occasionally during his days/evenings as a student. As an adult student in our CCE, Ron worked full-time while plowing through his schoolwork. When Ron graduated, we stayed in touch. Ron continued his job while looking for a change after receiving his diploma. He tells the story of running into his high school football coach. The coach inquired what Ron had been up to since returning from the Army. Ron told him about his experience at Guilford, his job, and his desire to get into something different. The coach had left the teaching and coaching profession and was working full-time as an insurance agent. He suggested Ron might want to give that a try. Ron took the bait and launched what has turned out to be an amazingly successful career. I won't take the time or space here to go into that journey, only to say that the shy, reserved Ron that I met in my office those many years ago took an entry-level job as an insurance agent and morphed into a nationally connected professional in the insurance and financial planning industry.

Becky and I were one of his first clients. I'll never forget how uncomfortable he seemed when he appeared at our door for the scheduled appointment. Little could either of us know then that forty years later, with both of us retired now, our friendship would develop as it has over those years. We don't see each other often. We talk frequently about our grown kids, his golf life, and my life as a man growing old and still trying to find the compass. I am so proud of the life had, and his wife have built. Both professionally and personally, Ron is a mentor and role model like few I have had the privilege to know and be able to call a dear friend.

One of the most lasting and impactful decisions Becky and I made during the first fifteen years at Guilford was the decision to move again. This time we would return to the site of Becky's growing up. She had grown up on a cow and tobacco farm. She lived in a one-story ranch house on Hastings Hill Road, less than a mile from where she graduated from high school. Her parents built that house themselves. They built it themselves with their own hands and tools. They would sell tobacco in the fall and buy materials. They would work all winter and go as far as the weather and the materials would take them. They would then do what farmers do the next spring, summer, and fall. Then the cycle would repeat until the house was done and Becky, her parents, and her brother could move out of the farmhouse they had shared with her grandparents for the first ten years of her life. The two-story traditional farmhouse (built in 1914 by her grandfather, Bunyon Smith) was located just behind and to the left of the new house. The two houses shared a driveway.

When Becky's grandfather Bunyon passed away, the old farmhouse became vacant. His second wife, Obera, had died earlier. The house stayed empty for a couple of years. Becky and I often talked over the years about whether it would be nice to build a house somewhere on the farm property one day. Becky's parents had made it clear they would welcome such a development and would make land available. (They had already done so for her brother Stan.) Well, we offered a variation of that plan. We asked if we could work out a deal to buy the old farmhouse and try to bring it back to life. I'll always remember Becky's mother immediately responding, of course. She asked if we wanted to tear it down and build a new house on the hill where it stood. After all, it was an old run-down farmhouse needing major repair and updating. We said "no." We wanted to resurrect it and make it livable once again. (In hindsight, I have often wondered if we made the right choice. As noted earlier, I have almost no mechanical skills and am totally inept at the fixing, repairing, etc., required to do what was needed.) But, take it we did. We did have to borrow $50,000 at the outset to bring it up to where we could get insurance. We had to put it up on jacks and replace roughly a third of its brick foundation. We had to update the wiring and plumbing and some heating. We had to build a two-story bathroom and closet addition. Most of that we hired out.

Some of it I did myself. I have joked with friends that I learned a lot about 2-inch putty. Nothing is plumb or square in a (now) 118-year-old farmhouse. There have been many times when I have wished we had said "yes" to Peggy. I am grateful we raised our kids in that environment, around industrious grandparents in that farm culture. They both learned something about the value of hard work and open spaces that was good for them to learn. I regret we did not have the resources to do more to the house sooner and with more professional workers doing the work. I was often embarrassed when I would see where the kids' friends came from and compared it to where my kids called home. I have never gotten over that. I still suffer from that comparative shortcoming. You see the recurring theme here. I can't help it.

Becky reminds me that the damage to our children must not have been too bad. When our daughter and her husband bought their first house in Clinton, MS, they purchased one built in 1884 in a historical section. That was their choice. They seemed to enjoy the work, treating it as a "work in progress."

Those first fifteen years on staff at Guilford went by quickly. I didn't think so then, particularly during the dark moments and days. (Time again.) The fact I still remember those times so vividly suggests that they are still too real in my psyche. Therein lies the truth. I still find myself succumbing to the memories. Yes, there are some good memories of some of those times. I would like to focus more on those. The pervasive memories of the failures, the stumbles, and the unrealized dreams are just too powerful and never-ending. I want to see Becky standing at the top of that gangplank. Instead, I see myself hiding in the bathroom stall while the association officers read my resignation letter and decide how to respond. Alas, time moves on. We are in the old farmhouse. The kids grew up with entirely different interests and skill sets. My faith walk continues to be central to the evolution of the story. It is hard to describe its progression.

The most significant takeaway from these years is that I consciously felt like a man on a mission, particularly related to my workdays. I was keenly aware of what a Guilford experience could do. I felt blessed to be a part of that experience and able to use my background as teaching fodder. My job was to enable families to afford that experience. I think my staff and I did that well. My real contribution was kissing Big Mouth Frogs and seeing where that might lead.

"Maybe There's a Mission Here." Maybe that heading was a little premature. I was thirty years old when I reported to work at Guilford. Perhaps somewhere in the deep recesses of my mind was the notion there was a mission calling me. Before getting the job at Guilford, I remember thinking I would like to return to my alma mater to close out my career when I got older. It would be an excellent way to say "thank you" to the institution that gave me more than my fair share of opportunities to succeed. It hadn't occurred to me that I might get there early in my professional life and spend three decades there. So, maybe there was a sense of mission then. Mostly, I was proud that I would be the Director of Financial Aid at Guilford College, my alma mater.

Those first fifteen years on staff at the college capture the essence of my story- an unexpected opportunity to begin again and get it right this time. It marked my real escape from The Project. I was young with a beautiful and talented wife and a growing family. No more changing direction every two to three years. No more falling short and having to struggle to right the ship. I was on my way. And so it was for the first few years. Then, as always, time caught up with me and my innate ability to ignore reality and not-so-blindly go where I knew better than to go.

I have always both craved attention and shunned the limelight. I wanted to be seen and recognized for my accomplishments while avoiding the spotlight and "settling for" invisibility. I always lived in the shadows of my best friends and work colleagues, even at family functions, withdrawing into a quiet and obscure presence. Professionally, early on, I had the ability to be well-liked. (Back to that Best Personality curse from high school.) I soon gained recognition as a new leader among financial aid colleagues across the state and even at the regional level. I didn't seek it. But it came. It came well before I had grown sufficiently in my new professional and personal world to be prepared to deal with it. I found myself accepting responsibilities I was ill-prepared to perform. I was making promises I could not keep. Suffice it to say, in a flash, my rising star disappeared from the sky because of my poor choices and resulting harmful acts. The new career, seemingly having just begun, was in jeopardy.

A career opportunity that had, just a short time earlier, looked like the path to the professional promised land, and a social revival suddenly became a place I had to go to every day to make a living. I did not get fired- but every waking minute, whether at work or home, for the longest time, I felt like I was suffocating from the feeling of shame and isolation I had brought upon myself. I would never again be a part of the financial aid family outside my immediate network at the college and a couple of friends in the business. I spent most of the next several years with my nose to the grindstone at work and trying my best to make up to Becky and the college for my failure- again. Gradually, the years went by. There's that ever-present demon again- time.

Chapter 17

SOMETHING NEEDS TO CHANGE

As MY CAREER at Guilford unfolded, particularly considering my previously disclosed professional isolation, I found myself focusing on two things- working whatever hours were required to do the very best job I could do and trying to be as good a husband and father as I knew how to be. This meant working long days, even pulling some all-nighters at high volume times in the financial aid cycle. It also meant staying late at work to pick Courtney up at dance classes several nights each week. We enrolled Courtney in gymnastics classes when she was little. She took to it like a duck to water. She was pretty good and competed at a high level by the time she was 12 years old. Then, as little girls often do, her body began to change. She grew taller, and her center of gravity changed, making many gymnastics maneuvers far more difficult. Her favorite part of gymnastics was the floor routine. When she came home from a meet where this realization became apparent, she told us she wanted to drop gymnastics and devote her time to dance. Her instructor in the gym for the floor routine was a dancer who ran her own dance studio. So, we went from getting Courtney to the gym a couple of times a week to getting her to the dance studio four to five times a week.

Lisa Kidd's studio, Arts Evangelica, became Courtney's second home. Becky and I would carpool from WCA to downtown Greensboro three or four nights a week and many Saturdays. I found myself staying at the office multiple nights a week. It didn't make sense to drive from Guilford College to High Point to downtown Greensboro, then home to Kernersville, only to turn around and drive back to Greensboro and then back to Kernersville. There was always work to be done at the office. So, that became a frequent routine. I didn't mind. Becky and I enjoyed watching Courtney grow in this arena. And, the Christian culture she was experiencing, both at Wesleyan and now at Arts Evangelica, was a good thing. The benefits were worth the price. That experience would direct Courtney's path for years to come.

The one downside of those choices was my being away from home so often at night. I've previously commented about a few memories of my father. I now believe I failed Scot in a similar way. I did not walk out on him and my family. We shared the house, time in the car, meals, and trips. But I was away from home during waking hours far too often. I don't know how I might have managed that time better. Just as I am grateful for the time Scot and I had together when I went back to college when he was six months old, I am equally sad that I failed to recognize and find a way to manage better that time during his teenage year. I cannot go back and recapture any of that time. None of us can. I cannot rid myself of the disappointment of knowing I failed as a father during those critical years.

That said, those years were not dull. Scot was doing well at Wesleyan. The school's ability to work around and outside some normal parameters to meet students where they were was precisely what Scot needed. To do so within a sound

Christian culture was what we were seeking. Wesleyan tried hard to find that happy medium between commitments to a serious Christian faith culture, a vigorous pursuit of academic excellence, and a genuine interest in putting forth an array of competitive athletic programs. We were pleased. Scot and his good friend (to this day) David Hunt co-authored a novel, "The Witch's Rite." It was never published, although I believe it could be, perhaps with some re-writing that comes from the years since then. Scot could take a class at Guilford and have it meet one of his Wesleyan requirements. Overall, it was a good mix. Courtney pursued her dance with a passion. She moved from the public school to WCA in fifth grade. As Lisa Kidd's Arts Evangelia grew and developed, so did Courtney's love of the dance.

When it came time to find a home for Courtney's sixteenth birthday trip abroad, I asked her where she wanted to go. To my surprise, she said, "Kenya." While Becky and I were on board with the going abroad plan, neither envisioned sending our sixteen-year-old daughter to Kenya- by herself. But we did. Again, through my Quaker connections at the college, I contacted a family in Nairobi. I knew the two children who had attended Guilford. The father was a government official, and the mother was a college educator. Where did Kenya come from in Courtney's thought process? Well! One of her favorite dance instructors was an African American young woman, Tina Yarborough. Courtney had taken several classes with her, some specifically African native dance. She loved it.

Without any accompaniment, Courtney flew to Nairobi, changing planes in Germany. I cannot imagine putting my sixteen-year-old daughter on such a journey in today's climate. She spent the first week in Nairobi. She was given an eye-opening tour of the city. She came home with a view of poverty she had never seen and few Americans ever see. She talked about seeing homeless children cooking chicken necks in tin cans over open street fires. After the first week, the family took its summer vacation to their" summer home" out in the bush. By Kenyan standards, it was an upper-middle-class family, wealthy enough to have a summer home and a live-in house girl. The summer home, a thatched roof abode, had no running water. The family did employ a house girl to fetch water from a well and, among other duties, prepare Courtney's bath for her at night. The dichotomy was not lost on Courtney at her young age. To this day, she is reluctant to walk into a department store and pay ridiculous prices for a sweater or dress. That six-week experience forever influenced her sense of priorities and life choices.

During this time, we discovered a new church home, of sorts. For a while, we had been unchurched. However, we regularly watched Robert Schuller's "Hour of Power" on tv. We parked on the living room couch every Sunday for a couple of years. While we were not engaged in a local congregation, we knew our kids were getting a proper faith-walk exposure at Wesleyan. Being actively involved in a local church would have been a better situation, but that was not the case, at least not until Courtney led us there.

Across the street from the campus of Wake Forest University in Winston-Salem sits what was then known as the First Assembly of God Church. Today it simply goes by Winston Salem First. In those days, and for many years before then, the church produced high-level Christmas and Easter theatrical productions. Many church members were drawn to the church because of its commitment to these productions.

Folks from across the Triad would come to see them. Their music and acting quality was impressive for an amateur production. That is how our family was introduced to First Assembly. Arts Evangelica was invited to participate in an Easter program. Some of Lisa's dancers would be angels in various stations. A small number, two or three, would dance on the top of the Tomb during the resurrection sequence. Courtney was selected to be one of those angels.

We enjoyed the program and seeing our daughter do what she loved in such a magnificent setting. I thought nothing more of it. I didn't know that Courtney was making friends with young people at the church. You guessed it- before long, Courtney wanted to attend their Sunday evening youth group. Next, she wanted to go to church there on Sunday mornings. I wound up taking her on Sundays. I would drop her off and get coffee and a Sunday newspaper. Before too long, curiosity got the best of me. My Quaker background was sure I would not be "at home' in this evangelical setting. And initially, that was right. But something happened along the way. When I first started attending, I sat in the back so I could leave without drawing attention. Soon, I found myself moving forward in the pews. After several weeks I was only ten-fifteen or so rows from the front. (This was a large church, seating probably 1500-2000 people when full). Then, one Sunday, something happened that I did not understand then and still not entirely today.

One of the morning's first congregational songs was "Surely the Presence of the Lord is in This Place."

Surely the presence of the Lord is in this place
I can feel His mighty power and His grace
I can hear the brush of angel's wings

I see glory on each face
Surely the presence of the Lord is in this place.
In the midst of His children, the Lord said He would be
It doesn't take very many
It can be just two or three
And I feel that same sweet Spirit that I've felt so many
times before
Surely, I can say I've been with the Lord.
Surely the presence of the Lord is in this place
I can feel His mighty power and His grace
I can hear the brush of angel's wings
I see glory on each face
Surely the presence of the Lord is in this place.
There's a holy hush around us as His glory fills this place
I've touched the hem of His garment
I can almost see His face
And my heart is overflowing with the fullness of His joy
I know, without a doubt, I've been with the Lord.
Surely the presence of the Lord is in this place
I can feel His mighty power and His grace
I can hear the brush of angel's wings
I see glory on each face
Surely the presence of the Lord is in this place.
Oh, surely the presence of the Lord is in this place!

I cannot explain what happened that morning. When the refrain "*I can feel His mighty power and His grace. I can hear the brush of angel's wings*" came up the second time, it was as real as anything I have ever experienced. I could *feel* the brush across my face. I didn't understand it then, and I don't understand it now. Something touched me that morning. No one will ever convince me I imagined something that morning, that I was merely "caught up" in the emotion of the moment. No- it was as real as if someone stood beside me and gently stroked my face with their palm. From that day, Becky, Courtney, and I became active participants in the ministry of First Assembly. Scot was in college by then and made his own choices in such matters. Even after Courtney went to college, Becky and I continued at First Assembly for several years, eventually leaving to return to the church of her youth. Suffice it to say these years encompassed a significant time in my faith walk. At one point, after hearing a visiting pastor talk about fasting and recounting his experience in lengthy fasting, I was led to undertake such an experience. This happened when Courtney was looking at colleges in the fall of her senior year at Wesleyan.

I will always remember a road trip to look at Hope College in Holland, MI- one of a handful of such road trips. I was 10-12 days into a 40-day true fast. I was hydrating and eating nothing. About that time, I did start drinking a little fruit juice from time to time. During our visit to Hope, we attended a group session for prospective students and parents. At some point, the leaders divided the group and took the students one way and the parents another. I decided to stay in the room where we had all gathered. At one end of the room was a buffet table laden with coffee, juice, and an array of fruits and pastries. For what seemed like an eternity, I paced in that room with one eye on that table and one eye on the door. For the better part of an hour, I lingered. Finally, I left the room, fast still intact. I knew then I could "do this." I knew then God was speaking to me through my commitment to be obedient and listen. I have never felt so close to God as I did during those forty days. I wish I could say that feeling persisted over the years. Had it done so, I wouldn't be recounting these memories and experiencing this dilemma now.

While at it, I should share Courtney's college decision and how that came about. After the series of road trips in the fall of her senior year, Courtney was unsure where she wanted to go. Then, in March of that year, she got a phone call from an admission counselor at Belhaven College (now University) in Jackson, MS. She had applied there early on and still needed to follow up on it. She wanted to major in dance, preferably at a school with a Christian culture. She had heard about Belhaven from Keith and Kathy Thibodeaux. Keith and Kathy founded Ballet Magnificat, a professional Christian dance troupe with a school in Jackson. Their cast came to perform in the Triad through contact with Lisa Kidd. The company relied on homestays to manage the budget. We were blessed to have the Thibadeaux stay in our home for two nights. During the visit, they made it a point to recommend Belhaven.

Sometime after that visit, the call came from the counselor at Belhaven. That call spoke volumes to me- just from a professional performance standpoint. The counselor was calling to follow up on Courtney's application. He noted she had not responded to any follow-ups and was simply curious why not. He hoped to understand so he (and staff in general) could learn how they might better convey their message in the next recruiting cycle. Courtney told him she liked what she had heard and seen in their literature; however, she wanted to major in dance, and all they had was a minor/concentration. The counselor listened and then asked her if she would consider at least coming to look in person and talk to some of the dance faculty if he told her she could be in the first class to major in dance. Yes- they would offer a dance major beginning with the class coming next fall. Before I knew it, Courtney and I were in the car heading to Jackson. After 48 hours of walking, looking, and listening, we were back in the car on I-20, coming home. Before we left the city limits of Jackson, I spoke to Courtney. I told her it was time to decide. It was March, and I was not driving to any more colleges. What did she think about this one? With no hesitation, she said, "This is it." I immediately launched into my college admin mode. I pointed out that the physical plant left something to desire in contrast to other places we had visited. Its performance venue was a dilapidated barn in comparison. Its campus-wide fiberoptic network was modest at best. I went on. When I finished, she responded, "It just feels right." I am a fortunate father to say neither of our children had ever given us a reason to mistrust their judgment. That was enough for me if it "just felt right" to her. The rest is history. Belhaven is where she spent the next four years, where she met her husband (a local two years ahead of her at Belhaven). Since then, Jackson and its surroundings have been home to Courtney and her family. She has now lived in Mississippi longer than in North Carolina. Becky and I joke it never occurred to us we would know our way around parts of central Mississippi as we do. You go where you must to share time and space with those you love.

What a journey- from gymnastics to dance, First Assembly, Belhaven. By this time, Scot was finishing his time at Guilford, having spent a whole year in Japan on a study abroad program. He loves Asian art, history, and culture- specifically Japanese. He returned to Japan after graduating from Guilford to teach English for a year, quite a different experience than his year there as a student. His year as a student was in Tokyo, attending The American University and engaging with Japanese and numerous international students. The year after college, he worked in the JET Program, teaching English to elementary-grade students in a small village on the northernmost island of Hokkaido.

The reader might have noticed that when I wrote about Courtney's college search and our road trips, I did not mention Becky's participation in those trips. Becky could not join in on those adventures due to her work schedule. Becky returned to school to secure her BS in nursing. Back then, most nurses were R.N.s, having graduated from three-year nursing programs, often hospital affiliated, rather than four-year college BSN degrees. By the time the mid-90s arrived, Becky was feeling the urge to up the credential. After taking required refresher courses, she enrolled in a year-and-a-half process at UNC-Chapel Hill while working full-time. She arranged her work schedule to be able to commute to Chapel Hill two days a week for that year and a half. She blew the top off it, getting her BSN from UNC. I was so proud of her. I always have been. This accomplishment was just one of so many reasons I have loved her these fifty years. Years later, she enrolled at Duke in their graduate school to obtain her MSN. In her late 60s, she did this while working full-time as a nursing instructor at Rockingham Community College. I could not be more proud of my wife.

Along with that pride comes the ugly head of the demons that never seem to give up. I look at her and wonder how much I have held her back professionally, socially, and financially. I look at her brothers. They are both terrific men, high achievers in their professions- the Navy and banking. I may be biased. In my opinion, Becky is the sharpest tack in that family box. Yet, after fifty years with me, she has nowhere near the financial security either of her brothers has. That is my fault, and I cannot change that. Now approaching my mid-70s, I regret nothing more; that

I failed to live up to my potential, specifically as it relates to preparing better for our later years. She deserves better—nothing I can do about it now. I am so sorry, Becky!

Something Needs to Change- that was the title of this chapter. As you have read, these years, essentially 1993 to 2008, were years of growth and change in family and work dynamics. Somewhere along the way, I began to feel a tug. It must have been in the mid-'90s. I wanted to sell Christian-theme t-shirts. They were coming of age then. I had two encounters that stoked the notion. Attending a Greensboro Bats minor league baseball game, I saw what appeared to be a young couple with, I assumed, their early teenage son. The kid was wearing one of those "Co-Ed Naked" t's. This one was Co-ed Naked Firefighters; "Find 'em hot… leave 'em wet." I couldn't believe what I was seeing. I thought, "And we wonder why kids do the things they do." What kind of message was this his parents were allowing? Sometime later, not sure just how soon, I was entering a K-Mart store at lunch one day. As I entered, a woman was leaving, wearing an oversized white t-shirt with black lettering that said, "DON'T ASK ME TO DO A DAMN THING." Again, I thought- what kind of message is this? I entered a period of research. I was sure there was a market for a brand of Christian t-shirts, not only citing Jesus as the genesis of the message, but also promoting a more positive attitude toward life in general.

I spent countless hours, days, and months, exploring this notion. Years passed, and I did nothing more than occupy time "researching." I never printed or sold a single shirt, post-it note, calendar, or whatever. The years went by. This was not the first time I was full of an idea and void of any action to bring it to life. This push and pull between ideas, dreams, and action and production has been a lifelong dilemma. This internal battle has never been more profound than during this period in the 90s and into the 2000s.

All was not lost during this period. There were some bright spots. In 2005 I had the honor of escorting down the aisle DeAnn Ingram, Courtney's best friend for many years. Courtney and DeAnn met when they were seven. Through gymnastics and dance, they became the best of friends. They worked on their crafts together. Courtney competed in and won the Junior Miss Forsyth County Pageant. DeAnn won the Junior Miss Randleman title. We vacationed together a couple of times. The irony is that our families never lived closer than forty minutes to each other and never attended the same school or church. However, they spent hundreds of hours together at the gym and then the dance studio and travel with the dance team. They were, and over the years into adulthood, are the best of friends. On one of those vacations at Myrtle Beach, DeAnn came to me one evening after everyone else had gone to bed. She wanted to ask me something. She had already spoken to Courtney to get her permission. Would I walk her down the aisle when she got married? Her father had not been a presence in her life since she was small. Her mother would "give her away" at the altar. She wanted me to walk with her. As I write these words, I can hardly hold back the tears. Rarely has anyone honored me so. I love DeAnn like a daughter. I was there in the hospital for 18 hours when her son was born. She has been a blessing.

The year ended in what is, without question, the darkest time of my life. I thought I might lose the love of my life. Our family on Becky's side always came together for major holidays. As was customary, we would all go to Uncle Burr and

Aunt JoAnn's mountain house near Sparta, NC, in the High Meadows Country Club community. That year was no different. But it was. Becky didn't feel well in the morning when it was time to make the drive. She insisted we all go on without her. Reluctantly, we did. She was sure she just had a stomach bug. We went on and had a great family Christmas gathering. Christmas had been a few days prior, but it was convenient to have these family events after Christmas.

Phone coverage in the mountains was sparse. I could not get a call out to Becky, and I did not hear from her. I assumed all was OK. When the food, the Secret Santa, and all the season sharing were done, and it was time to return to K'ville, we packed the car and headed down the mountain. Part of the way down the mountain, my phone rang. It was Becky. She had been trying to reach me and couldn't get through. She was having severe stomach pains. She was in a bad way. All the family was with us in the mountains, so she had no one else in the family to call. She did not want to call anyone else. I told her we would get there as quickly as we could. I was driving. It's a little over an hour's drive. I made short work of it.

When I entered the house, I knew we needed to immediately get her to the hospital. It was about a 10–12-minute drive to the ER. You know what came next. It took forever to be seen. If there was no blood, visibly broken bone, or apparent heart attack, you took a back seat in their triage formula. Finally, after what seemed like an eternity, a doctor did see us. With whatever evaluation they did, they could see no reason to keep her. They sent us home with something for the pain, not explaining what was causing the pain. We went home and tried to ease her pain. It only got worse.

I don't remember how long we stayed at the house. At some point, I decided we were going back to the hospital, and somebody was going to do something. I could not stand to see Becky in the kind of pain she was experiencing. She is a tough kid, always has been. I knew if she was expressing the hurt like she was, she was in severe pain and had to have some relief. Fortunately, this time she was seen quickly. She was admitted to a room, and the staff did everything they could to seek out the problem. The doctor was puzzled. She exhibited signs of appendicitis, but the X-rays showed no sign of an appendix. He came in to ask her when her appendix had been removed. She told him she had never had it removed. She had some "female" surgery years before. Could the surgeon have removed her appendix then? Not likely without her knowledge and consent. The doctor left to consult and ponder. I don't remember exactly the events that followed, only that Becky continued to writhe in pain. After a while, the doctor returned with the news. Her appendix had not been removed in surgery. It had recently burst, not a minor rupture; a massive burst. He had been led to think it had been removed because the X-rays showed nothing where the appendix should be. Her appendix had utterly exploded, and her body was now filling with poison exuded from that rupture. She was a sick woman and in a dangerous state. She was taken to surgery as soon as they could make the arrangements. They must clear the debris from the rupture and remove as much poisonous matter as possible. By now, her body and bloodstream were in a state of sepsis. She could die. I have never been more fearful of anything in my life. I stayed at the hospital night and day. I could not imagine the pain she was experiencing. I could not imagine my life without Becky in it. I don't remember how long she was in the hospital. I know it was several days before the doctor could tell us he thought she was "out of the woods." It was several more days before she felt like she had left the woods. Eventually, she did recover, and we returned home. Family and friends had taken down Christmas decorations. I hadn't given them a thought.

Thinking back on those days, I have to look ahead to the days to come. We are both in our seventies now. We both come from stock that has good longevity. It cannot be lost in my mind, though, that one or the other of us will face that time again-dealing with the loss of the one we love more than life itself. I am so grateful I did not lose Becky then. The peaks I have experienced, since and before, have almost all included her. As I write this, we recently shared a two-week road trip to Alaska to celebrate our fiftieth wedding anniversary. Just sharing time and space with that "cutest student nurse" I have ever seen is all I need nowadays. I pray for nothing more.

An unexpected peak during this period came a few years earlier, in the late 90s. One day, I got a phone call from Ken Nunn, a high school classmate. Ken was working on a class reunion of our high school Earthquakes football team. Ken was a leader on those successful teams and had been a good steward in keeping the group together. He drew upon his connections as a local Postmaster and career postal service guy to keep current address information. Somehow, in our conversation, the question, "What have you been up to" came about. I was not prepared for the response. Ken had just returned from a two-week volunteer church mission trip to Israel. Ken was not a real in-your-face hell-raiser in high school. He was not one I would have seen volunteering to do any Christian mission work in Israel. This was not his first trip and would not be his last. Ken told me about the trip and what he and his group did.

A former banker in South Carolina had quit his job, sold much of his belongings, obtained credentials, and moved to Peta Tikvah in Israel to build a baseball and a softball field complex. His plan, as he felt called to implement, was to create a facility where young people from all over Israel could come to learn the game of baseball. A Baptist retreat and conference center there pre-dated the birth of modern-day Israel. They welcomed this effort and offered the land. Ken and his group went to perform some routine annual maintenance and upkeep the ministry budget could not otherwise provide. After hearing the story, I asked Ken if he would go again. He said he would, and he would let me know when. I was blown away. I told him I would love to go when he went again. I told him I was not a Baptist but could be one for a few weeks if necessary. We both laughed. To my surprise, two years later, Ken called, and I was off to Peta Tikvah with a group of about a dozen men and women to work on a baseball complex. There was nowhere in Israel to purchase baseball equipment. So, we all were asked to take any equipment we could secure- new or used. The baseball coach at Guilford College, Nick Black, donated two sets of gently used catcher's gear, several bats and balls, and nearly a complete set of used uniforms.

We spent two weeks working and traveling around the country, escorted by in-country Baptist missionaries. It is impossible to describe those two weeks. You had to be there. Having spent much of my early adult life in the Quaker church, I had never been baptized. There, in Israel, I was baptized in the Jordan River by a Baptist missionary who, in his former life, had been a finish carpenter. How appropriate?

Years later, when I "retired" from Guilford, Becky and I went back- sort of a "close one chapter and open another" trip. I wanted her to experience the feeling of walking the steps where Jesus walked, seeing the terrain he observed, and feeling the Presence in a way you cannot feel any place else in this world.

When I returned from my trip to Israel with Ken and company, I was well on my way to a decision I had been mulling over for some time. The t-shirt idea had yet to grow legs. It never went anywhere. I finally concluded that was because that was not what God had called me to do. I had no experience in anything to do with selling T-shirts. By this time in the late 90s, I did have nearly thirty years of working with college kids and scholarships. Somewhere along the way, I began to think less about selling t-shirts and more about something else; a different calling. Perhaps God never intended for me to sell t-shirts, Christian or otherwise. Maybe He meant for me to use my talents and experience to "promote positive life choices" among a cadre of college-going Christians, college-going Christian artists and athletes. By the time 2008 came around, I had decided. We launched Motvation Ministry. I did all the legal work to create the 501c 3.

I put together the Board of Directors. I raised a little money and brought in the first class of Motvation Scholars in the fall of 2009, having worked the program part-time the previous year while still full-time at Guilford. Becky and I talked and prayed about it. She was unbelievably supportive of my decision. In April of 2009, I notified Randy Doss, my boss at Guilford, I would retire on October 15th, marking 30 ½ years at Guilford. It would be a financial struggle as I was not yet eligible for Social Security. I could begin to draw on my retirement, and if all went according to plan, I should be able to start drawing some salary from the ministry within two years. Little did I know what was to come; the impact of the real estate and stock market fall in 2008, my lack of success in fundraising, and my continued struggle with a sense of failure and comparative value.

As 2009 ended, I was excited about what lay ahead. Becky and I had a marvelous trip to Israel and Egypt. We returned and I hit the ground running. As far as I could see, I had no hint that much of my running would be "in place" with little meaningful results. Sitting here, writing this in mid-October 2022, I cannot find the words to describe the feeling of utter failure. When I talk with friends about this time, this experience, this effort, they all tell me I shouldn't feel this way; I can't know what I experienced was a failure. Perhaps I did not realize *my plans*, but maybe I did just what God wanted me to do. I need help getting to that place.

What a few years! Way too much to fully unpack in the few pages allotted herein! As I have attempted to relive these years for this exercise, much more work is needed than I can recount here. Perhaps, when I finish this project, I will start over again and go into greater detail with each chronological period visited here. I don't know. I hadn't realized quite so vividly how much 'stuff' out there was calling me to revisit. This exercise has brought that 'stuff' to the surface in ways I have tried to forget or keep buried. This recalling and writing project I convinced myself to undertake after writing 'The Letter' has left me with more unanswered questions than I had when I started. Once again, is time trying to commandeer the storyline? A closer look at the failures, the disappointments, and the shortcomings, from

different vantage points, affects how I look back on those times and how I now perceive the relevant impact of those times, compared to the WOW moments, the successes, the peaks. Could I reassess the time and the relative nature of cause and effect? Oh- so many questions- just when I was beginning to see the end of this- whatever <u>this</u> is.

I must do this now. Until now, I have intentionally shied away from directing too much attention to religion, theology, or my faith walk specifically. I have mentioned it occasionally and talked around it. In speeding through these fifteen or so years recalled in this chapter, I cannot deny the centrality of that walk to the daily life experiences covered herein. I also cannot deny how angry and disappointed I have become- angry and disappointed at God and myself.

For most of these years, I knew what I believed, and my faith walk demonstrated that belief. I knew I frequently fell short of what I thought God's expectations were. I was homed in on a belief system I thought was right. That belief led to my walking away from a 30 ½ year career at a place and job I loved. Believing I was heeding God's call, I left that security and stepped out in faith. Or did I? Was I heeding God's call? Or was I still seeking to succeed? Was I still failing in my decades-old self-worth profile? Was Motvation Ministry more about me becoming the President of something that would gain recognition and a following than it was about me following God's lead and going about His work? In October of 2009, I knew the answer to those questions. Now... Time passes- at its own pace- and I'm not so sure.

Chapter 18

YET ANOTHER CHANCE TO BELIEVE

THE NEXT SEVERAL years ushered in a very different phase of life. When I retired from Guilford in October 2009, I was a 30-year veteran of that culture, that schedule, that routine of responsibilities, expectations, colleagues, and rewards. During the last several years of my Guilford experience, I found myself wandering in and out of my faith walk. I have mentioned the life-impacting experience at First Assembly. My 40-day fast early during that period did have a lasting impact on me. I was trying hard to shake those lifelong fears and feelings of failure and lack of value. Trying hard or not, I was not having much success. When I decided to retire and commit fully to building Motvation Ministry, I was convinced I was on the right path. I was convinced that taking that step would give me the courage and tools to succeed. I'd often heard the adage that God does not always call the equipped. He sometimes equips the called. I knew I was not equipped, even though I was a career college financial aid professional. I was being called to continue working with college students in a different capacity. With all my heart, I believed I was doing what God called me to do.

By this time, I had been involved with the Promise Keepers movement, attending several stadium functions- sometimes alone, sometimes with men from First Assembly. Later, after launching Motvation, I would connect with a local Christian men's group- the Winston-Salem chapter of the New Canaan Society. NCS is a non-denominational group that meets weekly for coffee, a devotional, a speaker, and genuine networking and sharing. The attendees are typically successful businessmen, with a smattering of NPO types like me. I found these group meetings a welcoming and loving place. I routinely heard stories from local or visiting folks who, like me, had responded to a calling to do God's work. Often, these stories included a recitation of the struggles and failures they had experienced.

Initially, I found this encouraging. However, as time went on, I realized I had never heard stories that paired with my experience as I moved through trying to build Motvation. After three or four years, I realized I was not building a sustainable ministry. By year three, I needed to raise more funds to continue to grow the scholarship pool, much less even begin to absorb the non-scholarship expenses associated with the enterprise. I was putting retirement savings into the ministry and not even close to drawing a salary. By year three of the launch, I was already back in a state of fear and failure. I thought I was answering God's calling and it was not working. At least, it was not working as I had anticipated. Friends tell me just because I did not have the experience I thought I would have does not mean God's plan was not being realized.

Let me back up a little bit. One of the peaks of my life was the day I left Guilford- not so much that I was leaving Guilford, but the way my boss, co-workers, friends, and students said "goodbye." I knew they were planning a send-off. Anyone with thirty years in the game was going to be recognized. I had already been asked whether I wanted my official

Guilford College chair to be with rockers or without. (I chose with). What I didn't expect was the turnout. I walked over to the Gilmer Room in the college caf and was greeted by a room full of Guilford folk. My wife and in-laws were seated up front. I was stunned to see several former students who came from hours away to participate in this event. These were students who, in some cases, had worked in our office. Others babysat our kids. One I had recruited on an admission recruiting trip, only to discover her parents were from my hometown. I cried like a baby at her wedding some years later. Three of these students worked in the financial aid business for several years- one, now, is a VP in Washington for the National Association of Student Financial Aid Administrators. I was overwhelmed by the show of appreciation and love. Rarely have I been so moved. Several people spoke briefly. At the conclusion, I could speak- to say "thank you" for a good ride and to talk about Motvation Ministry and what I felt I had "been called" to do.

I remember going home with Becky and thinking what a wonderful day I had just had. I was excited to get underway on my new adventure. I was not foolish enough to think there would be no failures and disappointments. I went home that night ready to wake up the following day and hit the ground running on what I thought would be my full-time endeavor for the rest of my working life. I could not foresee how short that trip would be.

Before telling more of the story of Motvation, I must share one more trip experience with Ken Nunn. After Ken and I had reconnected and shared time in Israel, he and I stayed in touch regularly. We still do. We didn't see each other often, but we did keep in contact. One night, I got a call from Ken with one of the strangest invitations I ever received. He wanted to know if I would be interested in being a Park Ranger for the US National

Park Service. What? What on earth was he talking about? OK-here's the story. Ken has been an avid national park enthusiast for some time. Somewhere along the way, he discovered Portsmouth Island off the coast of North Carolina. The island is a part of the National Park system. It is unusual as national parks go, however. It is a small, uninhabited island between Ocracoke and Cedar Island. There is no permanent Park Service presence there. During peak season and into the fall, the Park Service provides staff to open the buildings still on the island and welcome any tourists that might find their way there. Portsmouth Island was a crucial shipping point from the mid-1700s to the mid-1800s. A massive hurricane in 1846 created the Oregon and Hatteras Inlets, thus beginning the demise of Portsmouth as a necessary landing point for incoming or outgoing cargo.

By the mid-1950s, only twelve residents were still on the island. It is now totally uninhabited. There are a few buildings on the island: a school, post office, church, and other small commercial and residential buildings. In addition, there is the sight of the US Lifesaving Station, built in 1894. Visitors are mainly small groups interested in the island's unique history, or its current-day animal and floral wildlife. The Park Rangers, when staffed, are notified when the small boat service that ferries folk to the island has guests coming. The Staff meet these visitors at the dock, give them a brief history, and encourage them to wander the island at their leisure.

Well, that was the reason for the call. Ken had gotten into volunteering to be the Ranger on several occasions. He was calling to see if I would like to do it. The Park Service required two people to be present, given the location and seclusion of the site. It would be a three-week stint in mid-October. We would be the final staff in the park for that season. When our time ended, we would ensure everything was buttoned up and keys returned to the Park Service on Cedar Island. I was fascinated by the possibility. I have never been a national park enthusiast. This sounded interesting. Then, the "but" came. Ken explained there had to be two rangers on duty. I asked him who had done this with him previously. I believe his wife, Lucy, had been there, and his best friend from high school, Mike DeGrechie, had done it once. I forget who else had accompanied him. I asked about one of his previous guests doing it. Then, the rest of the story came out.

Ken gave me the rest of the scoop. There is no running water, bathrooms, or electricity on the island- other than in the small living quarters provided for the Rangers. That space is a small building next to the Lifesaving Station that served as its stand-alone kitchen when it was in service. The building had been divided into a kitchen, a sitting area, and a sleeping space with barely enough room for two people on single beds. The kitchen had a small gas stove and fridge. There was a gas heater about the size of a small microwave. Between the kitchen and sleeping quarters was the bathroom, barely big enough to sit down, with a shower stall just big enough to turn around it. Natural gas tanks provided the gas that had to be replaced regularly. The electricity came from batteries with a limited diesel backup. What Ken described was the most Spartan living conditions I had ever experienced. By mid-October, it gets frigid at night on an island barely a mile wide off the coast of NC. Ken and I would run the gas heater and describe how cold the night had been by how many bricks in the heater we had to heat up. Had it been a one-brick, two-brick, or three-brick night? There was no television. Cell phone usage was unreliable.

Bottom line- Ken could not get anyone who had been before to go back. Oh- I forgot to tell you. The place was mosquito infested. They were so thick you could see them in swarms. Fortunately, Ken had learned how to prepare and deal with them over the years. I said yes in a moment, somewhere between weakness and adventurous curiosity. I would do it. I won't take any more time here to relive those days. I did go back two more times.

I've taken some time to recall this episode for several reasons. This was so far outside my usual comfort zone. I am not a beach person, at all. I had no desire to spend three weeks "at the beach." I welcomed the opportunity to reminisce with Ken about our high school days. I had learned enough about his faith walk to believe I could benefit from some extended time with him. Those days at Portsmouth were informative both from a historical narrative standpoint and a personal inner-searching standpoint. The days and evenings provided time and space to be alone with my head and feelings in, what I believe, was constructive time. I am grateful to Ken for asking. While the occasional reflection on my pending dilemma had marinated for a few years, the notion that there might be more than a casual academic monologue taking place in my head began to take form during those days. It's motivational what solitude, mosquitoes, sand, and salt can do.

Here is where I planned to describe the birth, development, and death of Motvation Ministry during these years. In the context of this epistle, these years, and their aftermath, mark a critical period in my struggle with my self-image and faith walk. As reported previously, the decision to launch Motvation Ministry in 2008, after nearly fifteen years of hemming and hawing about what God was calling me to do, was a significant step for me.

Not only did it mean launching a tool that, hopefully, would positively impact the lives of numerous young college men and women. It also meant walking away from a thirty-year career at Guilford College- a place I loved, a place that had given me more than my fair share of opportunities. That also meant walking away from a safe financial status and future. I wasn't getting rich at Guilford, but I was financially safe. Leaving that safe place meant I would have no salary coming in, at least for a while. I was prepared for that. Becky and I discussed it and were good with the path forward. I never considered a Plan B. If I worked hard and was faithful to the plan, I could start drawing a salary in a couple of years and not have to continue to support the ministry from my retirement funds.

I have no idea if anyone will ever read any of this. I hope my children and grandchildren will someday. I do not want to cause them any pain, but these words will help them know and under-stand Dad (and Pappy) in a way and at a level they could never do otherwise. That said, the details of the Motvation experience are irrelevant. I may write about that in more detail in another effort- depending on the outcome of this exercise.

I want to address a couple of salient items about the program's launch and management. They are relevant to this process. When moving toward launching Motvation, I was convinced I needed a scriptural reference as the foundation for our work. I am no Biblical scholar, and I appreciate that one can justify anything with scriptural references. Nevertheless, I was committed to having a scriptural foundation for the work. After some considerable research, I settled on Philippians 4:8,9.

"8 Finally, brothers and sisters, whatever is true, whatever is noble, whatever is right, whatever is pure, whatever is

lovely, whatever is admirable—if anything is excellent or praiseworthy—think about such things. ⁹ Whatever you have learned or received or heard from me, or seen in me— put it into practice. And the God of peace will be with you." *NIV Version*

I chose this advice because it makes sense when thinking about a fundamental message to instill in these young people as they got up every day to pursue their long-imagined college experience, often amid a culture alien to their prior Christian experience. I knew from the data that an overwhelming percentage of church-raised Christian collegegoers leave the church during their college years, many during that first year. By associating them with a proper adult Christian mentor who could remind them often of this message, we could make a dent in that percentage. The scholarship money was merely a hook to get them to apply for our mentoring program. The mentoring connection was the real meat of our effort. This verse seemed to speak to the point; if these kids could teach themselves to get up in the morning and "think about such things" as they go about their day, they would be more likely to make better life choices during the day. When I talked to students, potential mentors, and others, I spoke about decision-making. None of us, including college students, roll out of bed in the morning and think consciously, "OK- what can I do to screw my life up today?" That's not what we do. All too often, we go about our days making choices/decisions that, in the moment, seem innocuous, or only minimally consequential at best. Any of them, in and of themselves, may be insignificant. The issue concerns the impact a string of bad choices, growing more extensive and more destructive, can have over time. One can think of any number of bad results from an action that had its origin multiple choices/decisions before the immediate choice that led to the harmful act. Our goal was to use the mentorship tool, based on the Phil 4:8,9 guidance, to help these young people make better choices during these challenging years. Again, no one consciously chooses in the morning to screw their life up today," but many will make a series of bad choices that can lead to that outcome. The mantra I shared ad nauseam, I am sure, was: **Friends- Choose them carefully! Choices- Make them wisely! Consequences- Embrace them graciously!** The strange place I find myself today is remembering and writing these words in the context of this exercise. *I don't know how to navigate the disconnect between these words of advice and my feelings, long-held and continuing to gnaw.*

When I first began to move on the notion of what would become Motvation Ministry, I focused on the generic college-going Christian student. Early in the process, I began to feel a need to narrow that focus. One of the many things I learned at Guilford was that students often arrived on campus with built-in skill sets and platforms. Athletes and artists specifically show up with such tools available to exploit. I decided to focus the work of Motvation on athletes and artists, hoping they would use their skill sets and campus platforms to spread the Phil 4:8,9 message, both in word and deed.

Each year, for enrollment periods from the fall of 2009 to the fall of 2012, we processed applications, selected ten recipients, funded scholarships, and arranged mentoring connections. Our original commitment was to fund 4-year scholarships to ten new recipients each year, building to a full cadre of forty Motvation Scholars each year. We hoped to begin adding to each new year's quota when we reached that level. By the time we reached the fourth year, it was clear our funding was not keeping up with the scholarship demands. We only funded part of the scholarship requirement with donor gifts. Even in the first year, when we only needed to fund $10,000, I had to put funds from my retirement account to meet that demand. I was not concerned. As we built the cadre and reached out to potential donors, I believed we would meet the financial needs, and I would not need to use my retirement resources. I believed donors would come forward to meet these growing scholarship needs and cover administrative overhead, even providing some reasonable income level for me. I knew when the time came to hire a replacement for me, some years into the future, we would need to pay for that. It made sense to build that into the budget early.

Those third and fourth years were difficult. I had not expected anything like what we were experiencing. As I mentioned previously, I had no Plan B. I knew I was heeding God's call and doing His work. I quickly realized what I already felt- I was not qualified to do this work. I had the skills and experience to administer the scholar selection process and procure mentors. What I should have done was devote more time, energy, and focus on defining and cultivating the mentor/scholar relationships. I spent too much time and focus trying to raise money, which was way outside my wheelhouse. I was asking people for money. Remember my father telling me not to ask him for anything? I have spent my entire life afraid to ask for anything. How could I pull this off, knowing it meant asking people for help and money?

I believed the adage that God would equip the called, not necessarily call the equipped. Moreover, this was terrible timing. I launched Motvation in 2008, during the catastrophic collapse of the housing market in the US and the near global economic collapse. Businesses were failing right and left. Start-ups were going under. It was no time to start a new business, much less a faith-based scholarship and mentoring program. Even though the focus of Motvation was mentoring, not scholarships, I had built it around a scholarship entrance tool, and I needed the funds and the fundraising acumen to see that through.

When it was time to launch the application cycle for the fall class of 2013, the board and I agreed to cancel the process for new applications. We would continue to fund current recipients to keep our original commitment. We were able to see that through for two more years. Our last scholarship checks were written for the spring of 2015, meaning we did not fund our final year's recipients through their entire four years.

I visited many scholars individually during their first year of college, and a few more often than that. I have stayed in touch with many of these fantastic young men and women. Most are now married and raising families of their own. Having to "lay down" this ministry and renege on the total four-year commitment to some is one of the most painful things I have ever experienced. As of this writing, it has been ten years since the decision to lay it down. After having to cease operations and after having invested roughly 20% of my retirement funds into the program, I have not had a day that I have not wondered how and why this happened. I have friends who tell me I should not think about this as a failure. I should think that perhaps we did precisely what God had planned for us. We cannot know his plans for us, or the impact our work had or will have on any of those kids and their mentors, not to mention their lives as they "pay it forward." I get all that. I am still angry about the financial cost and, once again, the feeling of utter failure and disappointment. I have spent my entire life, from my growing up days in Fairview Homes, to my in-and-out experiences as a student at Guilford College, to my working years at the college, and then to my post-Guilford "calling" trying to be relevant, trying to be good, and, yes, trying to make a positive difference. I found myself attending New Canaan Society meetings and hearing the amazing successes of Christian brothers who shared their stories of failure, disappointment, and destruction, telling how God had miraculously met their needs and enabled them to meet their challenges. I was increasingly less impressed and even more discouraged. If God had called me to build Motvation Ministry, knowing I was not equipped, why had He allowed me to fail to develop the skills to become equipped? How could I fall so short of becoming adequately equipped? Must I believe I was never "called" in the first place and pursued something I wanted to do for whatever reason? Or was I called to accomplish exactly what we did in the lives of the students we reached in that short period? If that is the case, why not just tell me so? Why would God allow me to leave behind a productive professional career, embark on a mission I thought I was called to pursue, and then let me fall short of the vision I saw, only to accomplish what He had in mind all along? This is all very confusing and dangerously evocative. Either way, I can't get beyond reliving those years and the sense of failure and disappointment. I am not a particularly good follower of the Phil 4:8,9 teaching I preached.

It is a little after 4:00 p.m. on a Wednesday in early November. Sitting in my office in Scot's bedroom, I can look

*outside a big north-facing window and see traffic heading
up the hill and curve across Salem Parkway). Now thirty-
some years after moving into 'this old house,' I occasionally
pause and think back on these years at the top of this hill. I
remember the two giant oak trees struck by lightning that
we had to have removed. That changed the landscape of this
entire hilltop. I think about beautiful snowy winter days
when I could look out back and marvel at the glistening
white pasture leading to the glass-topped pond, surrounded
by snow-covered branches of all types and sizes. I remember
walking with grandkids through the snow down to the Big
Rock at the south end of the property, then watching Abby
pause and take mental pictures on the walk back, putting
her make-believe camera to her face and snapping visions of
what she was seeing so she could take them with her back to
Mississippi- and wherever else her life takes her. I remember
dreading having to once again go into the tobacco fields and
barns to help Peggy and Royce as they went through their
annual ritual of planting, tendin' to, harvesting, drying,
and selling their crops. I remember Becky and I wanted to
raise our kids in this old house, then doing it. (I learned to
be careful what you wish for.) I remember watching Peggy
and Royce grow old. I didn't realize I was doing the same
thing at a later starting line. I miss Royce. In many ways,
he did become the father I never knew. I still spend time
with him. I take my walking stick with me when I go on
my walks. It is a small tree limb with a vine that grew
around and embedded itself into it. Royce found it and cut
it. After Royce died, I found it in the old tobacco packhouse
where Royce had stuck it. Royce was good at leaving things
lying around like that. I enjoy my walks with Royce. I miss*

seeing anyone in the house just up the driveway from our house. We had to move Peggy into an independent living facility nearly two years ago. She is 92 and her memory is fading. She still gets around well with her walker and has many friends. She is rapidly losing any memory of what happened earlier today or yesterday.

I could go on and on about what I remember, harking back to those growing-up days in Goldsboro. Why should I? If I have learned anything during this effort, it is that no matter where I find myself landing in this time parade, I cannot get away from the fact that time always commands the playing field. No matter what good times, WOW moments, or successes I may have encountered, time has managed to hasten its pace past those moments only to grind to a near halt at every valley, failure, disappointment, and shortcoming.

So, the years since Motvation launched have undoubtedly seen their share of good days. Many of those days were directly related to Motvation and its world. Other good days were much more important as Becky and I shared time and space as we are so wont to do. Still, others flow readily through my mind as I see Scot and Courtney becoming adults and following their chosen life paths. I grasp at those moments as I would for air to breathe. But they are just that-moments. I don't know why. Why must those times assume only momentary residence in my mind, while so many other times on the other far end of the spectrum occupy such an unfair share of my memory? Even now, sitting here gazing out the window onto Hastings Hill Road, why must I work so hard to focus on those moments, only to succumb to the devil that time becomes?

What started as an effort to reflect on "Yet Another Chance to Believe" quickly became another exercise in succumbing to time and its unrivaled ability to dictate the rules. I don't like these rules any more now than I did when we began this journey.

Chapter 19

DOES IT REALLY MATTER?

THIS MORNING I am sitting at the small dining table at the house in Black Mountain, NC. The house belongs to my son-in-law's father. He and Courtney are kind enough to allow Becky and me to come here to enjoy the leaves at this time of the year and give me something of a sanctuary amenable to this exercise. For several months now, I have been stymied in my efforts to conclude this process. Much like earlier, when I was trying to write past the time when I was in junior high school and was cut from my basketball team tryouts and my daddy walked out on the same night, I find myself having difficulty getting past another emotional roadblock. Having to lay down Motvation Ministry and all that went into that physical act and its emotional baggage has been utterly debilitating. That, coupled with the calls I received from my friend, Paul Coscia, to come help in the Financial Aid Office at Salem College, keep distracting me from the mission at hand. The fact I also am being forced to come to grips with my own physical mortality (aside from the circumstances at the heart of this epistle) has made bringing this exercise to a conclusion even more difficult.

I must confess though- I do miss Jethro. Oh, yes, about Jethro! Before getting into the meat of addressing the final years of this journey, I must introduce Jethro. Over the years, our family has enjoyed the company of several wonderful canine friends, starting with Fritz von Rasputin, who I introduced earlier. Growing up in The Project, we were not allowed such pets. I always wanted one. So, Fritz came into our lives early. Over the years, we had several other dogs of various and mixed varieties. When we had to put down our last dog, Jesse, due to cancer, I swore I did not want another "pet." Parting was just way too painful. Little could I imagine that, just like Jesse, another homeless, lost, four-legged critter would find its way into our home and hearts. This time it was of the feline persuasion. Little Jethro showed up at Becky's parents' house next door, a little-bitty kitten that fit in the palm of her hand, black with a white tuxedo and tummy with beautiful white pantaloons on all four legs. I wanted no part of a cat. I thought I was allergic to them.

Becky set out to find a home for Jethro, only to discover you cannot give away a kitten. Nobody would take him. Becky took him to the vet where we learned he was about five weeks old. He had a lung infection and only a 50% chance of surviving. I came around to thinking that we could allow him to stay if he survived, but he would have to be an outside cat. I could not have him in the house. Then, I made a mistake (not really a mistake) of reading up on stray kittens' survivability and learned that such cats living fully outdoors had a much shorter life expectancy, even more so when in a situation like ours- in the country with all kinds of natural predators and road traffic. After about eight weeks, I told Becky she could quit trying to find him a home. He could stay. Jethro (originally, he was to be called Mr. Gibbs after the star on Becky's favorite tv show- "NCIS") had stolen my heart. He had Becky from the beginning. It took me a few weeks to get aboard that train.

I tell you all this to explain what I mean when I say I miss Jethro. I do not understand many things in life- the comings and goings of people and events. I am trying to figure out what I think about miracles experienced and miracles unrealized. When I hear a believer say" God is good" when something good or miraculous occurs in their life, I want to ask, does that mean God's goodness is dependent on whatever good thing happens? So many questions. So little to fully KNOW! I DO KNOW that an unexpected and unwanted little five-week-old miracle came into my life the day Becky discovered him at the foot of the basement steps, meowing for all he was worth. He had to have fallen and tumbled down those steps. He was too small to have walked down them. He is now five years old. His head is bigger than his entire body when Becky found him. He has received regular vet care. We do our best to see he is well, nourished, and loved. When out of town, we hire a niece to come house(cat) sit, rather than board him at the vet.

It is not too much of an overstatement to say Jethro saved my life. Certainly, he saved my mental and emotional state. After losing Motvation, I wandered into a very dark place. I still struggle with it. As catalogued in this epistle, I have struggled to find joy, happiness, and meaning all my life. (Were it not for the love of my life, I do not know if I would have survived. I imagine few of my family, friends, and colleagues have ever known this aspect of me.) Then, along came Jethro. I have smiled and laughed more in the past four years than in any period I can remember since the first years of marriage. He has stolen our hearts. His go-to place every morning is Becky's lap. He ends my every night climbing up on my chest and looking right into my eyes. Then he settles onto my lap and commences to "bathe", then nap. I joke that I have become his favorite bathtub. When I get up each morning, he greets me with his morning "demand" that I pick him up and walk outside with him. After a brief look around the property, he lets me know he is ready to go back inside and straight to his treats jar. I follow his instructions. We play tag and hide & seek- all on his time and his terms. I laugh- something I have missed all too often. Sure, some moments bring laughter- those moments with the kids and grandkids, the occasional sporting event, etc. Rare has been the indwelling sense of joy that Jethro has unlocked. So, back to my initial comment when I began today's writing- I miss Jethro. I don't like to think about when he might no longer be a part of my life.

Back to the question at hand- "Does it really matter?"

Reflecting on the years since laying down Motvation and everything those years have encompassed, I have to say, "I don't know." My initial reaction is, "Does anything really matter?" My good friend, my Thursday morning breakfast buddy, Rev. Rick Lebaube loves woodworking. He loves to procure old wood pieces and make amazing things from them- furniture and accessories. Even with her full-time duties as a nursing instructor, Becky finds time to create beautiful one-of-a-kind handmade jewelry and incredible Ukrainian eggs. I see what they and others do, and I envy them. It is almost like when we buried Motvation, a part of me died also. Today, I can think of absolutely nothing that motivates me to want to "do" much of anything. That bothers me. I remember when my Papa lived with me and Mama and died in our apartment at age 84. I learned that he became bedridden years earlier, after the death of his second wife. I was told he just quit. He just gave up. He had lost all reason to live. So, he quit living and went to bed. I sometimes I think I understand.

That is not to say the years post-Motvation have lacked activity and movement; quite the contrary. About the time we buried Motvation, Becky changed jobs. Her nursing career had been in maternal-childcare and pediatric nursing, from labor & delivery to teaching Lamaze to home care specializing in working with extremely sick babies and children. She had often talked about perhaps teaching. Although she did not have the required Master's Degree, she applied for a teaching job at a local community college. Her breadth and depth of experience and her undergraduate B.S. from UNC were enough to get her an interview. That's all she needed. After being offered the job, she agreed to get her Master's. At the age of 65 she enrolled at Duke while still teaching full-time. Two and a half years later, she graduated with her Master's in Nursing Education. I cannot tell you how proud of her I have always been. That challenge and how she managed it only bolsters that pride even more. Even here, that angry demon rears its head. To be honest, I must admit I was jealous. While I watched her go about her daily work and then tackle the academic mission she had chosen, I felt so small in comparison. I found myself looking back at my failures.

Coming out of high school, I was an academic leader. I was a UNC Morehead Scholarship nominee. I didn't win the scholarship, but being a nominee was rarified air. Then, just two years later, I was a college dropout. How could that be? Then, three additional years later, I returned to college, got married, and dropped out again. After starting a family and finally graduating from Guilford, I started coursework pursuing a Master's in Public Administration on two occasions at two different universities. I didn't stay with it beyond a semester either time.

So, while I was, and am, immensely proud of the woman with whom I have been blessed to share my adult life, her successes serve to remind me of my failures. She shares no blame for this. If she ever reads this, I pray she will not feel discomfort in any way. My failure in preparation and performance in this regard was due in no way to her. She has always been more encouraging and supportive than I could have ever deserved.

A couple of years after Motvation, our son Scot turned forty. You may recall my earlier recounting our sending our kids to live abroad for six weeks during the summer of their sixteenth birthdays. Well, now it was time to celebrate Scot's 40th birthday. This time we would get to participate. We planned a ten-day trip to England, Paris, and Normandy. Scot is quite the WW II buff. On our budget, such a trip required considerable planning and saving. We were excited. We had tickets for the Royal Albert Theatre to see The Phantom of the Opera. We bought in advance tube and train tickets to get around London and other sites outside London. We had hotels booked in Paris and our trip to Normandy from there. Our first day in London was terrific. We spent a good portion of it in the British Museum. We toured Churchill's wartime command bunker. We returned to the tube station late in the afternoon to get to our hotel in time for dinner and the theatre. Just about a block from the tube station, walking on a cobblestone sidewalk, Becky tripped and fell. At first, we thought she had just hurt her wrist and mouth. She had hit her chin and broke a tooth. She immediately felt pain in her wrist. Moments later, as we tried to help her get up, she was in severe pain in her right shoulder. Becky has always had a high pain and discomfort threshold, perhaps from her farm background.

Scot and I managed to get her to the tube station, about a block away. By the time we arrived there, she was in trouble. The pain was increasing. Still, we had no idea the severity of the damage. We knew she had chipped a tooth and suspected she might have broken her wrist. We thought she might have dislocated her shoulder. Once inside the tube station, we were able to locate the station manager. The good news was the immediate attention and professionalism shown by the attendant in charge. He was able to offer some immediate, low-level first aid. Quickly, we all agreed that more assistance was needed than could be administered by us there on the floor of his office. He called for an ambulance. It seemed like forever before any help arrived. London is a big and crowded city. It took about thirty minutes before help arrived. And it was not an ambulance. It was a paramedic on a bicycle. Ambulances can't navigate the traffic in the city in any kind of timely fashion. Paramedics on bikes are the first course of response. (This may be the case in most large city environments). The paramedic was able to provide stronger relief medication. It was more potent, but still, Becky was in great pain. Even then, all Becky could say was she was so sorry for spoiling our day. I tried to assure her our day had not been spoiled. I was more concerned about her pain than any vacation event that had been interrupted. At that time, I did not know what was coming down the road and the magnitude of the interruption.

I don't know how long we were in the tube station with the paramedic and station manager before an ambulance finally arrived. It was quite a while. We were taken to the University Hospital, where we checked in to the emergency department-virtually no paperwork and no billing information as precedent for entry. I do not want to relive more of that event, so I will cut to the chase. After numerous attempts to draw blood (Becky has always been a difficult stick), staff took her for x-rays. When the doctor came in with the results, he asked, "Which is your dominant hand?" She replied, "My left." to which he responded, "Well, that's about all the good news I have for you." He showed us the picture. He said it looked like what you might see if you took a light bulb and tapped it against a wall. Her right shoulder had been shattered. It was in pieces. There could be no mending with screws.

A total replacement would be required. The staff took us to a room (no private room, a ward of four people-welcome to the British National Health Service). There she would spend the night to have surgery the following day. Becky and I immediately agreed we would fly home the next day and have the surgery here. We had to talk Scot into staying and finishing out the rest of the trip. It was all paid for and we did not have trip insurance, so there was no refund on anything we had paid (lesson learned). There was nothing he could do anyway. So, he did staid. I am glad. I got on the phone and booked a flight home the next day. When there was nothing more to do at the hospital, Scot and I returned to the hotel to pack for the morning. There I made two phone calls- one to my good friend, Rick LeBaube, and the other to Rev. Frank Thomas, my New Canaan brother. I cannot describe how much hearing and receiving their prayers meant, and still means, to me. These days, in my darkest hours, I think back on that experience and these brothers being there. I am forever in their debt.

The hospital bundled her up and gave her the most potent pain meds they could with sufficient dosage to keep her 'as comfortable as possible' for the long trip home. In the morning, when the nurse came to tell us we could leave, that was it. We received no bill. We did not have to stop by any discharge office or bursar. Likewise, they just said we could leave. We had to find a wheelchair and get help hailing a cab. Once they told us we could go, the staff offered no assistance in making that transition. Scot came and helped us maneuver so we could get to the airport. Even at the airport, there was virtually no assistance. Anyone could see we needed help- baggage and a woman obviously drugged and trussed up. But no offer of help. We did find our way to the correct terminal. The taxi driver had delivered us to the wrong stop. After a long flight, we landed in Charlotte. We immediately called the orthopedist Becky wanted to see. When she saw the doctor, he told us we had made the right decision. He would treat her with pain medications for several days before operating. After seeing the x-rays, he told us the worst thing we could have done would have been to have the surgery the day after the event. The tissues needed time to begin getting over the trauma of the injury before going in. Becky had the surgery, and it went well. Then, after several days post-surgery, she started a long and painful course of PT, both in the office and at home. I always knew I married a tough kid. I never saw it displayed quite like I saw it during those weeks. I can only imagine her pain during the flight from London. Never did I see her cry or show anger. For several weeks she had to sleep sitting in a chair. I shudder to think about the nights she had little or no sleep. I hope I never have to see my sweetheart in such pain again.

It was an expensive disappointment caused by no one. It was an accident. Accidents happen every day to good people and bad. No one died. Sometimes they do when accidents occur. So, I understand the relative significance (or insignificance) of the events of that time. That understanding, however, does not reduce the reality of my sense of disappointment. Once again, a much-anticipated peak experience was dashed and turned into another painful memory. Most of the peak moments I have experienced over these past 50 years have directly involved Becky specifically, and my extended family indirectly. This turned out not to be one of those times, not solely because our long-planned trip was scratched, but because of the pain and suffering I saw the woman I love endure. She blamed herself for what happened. It was just an accident- no one's fault.

From the time of that truncated vacation trip to today, a few other life stories have taken place. Before bringing this epistle to a close, I should share some of them, not because they have any great lasting value; but they have occupied my time these past few years. Given my state of mind, someone other than me is the one to gauge their value.

One of the most important changes in our lives during these past few years was our move from church membership and attendance at First Assembly of God in Winston-Salem, which had been at the core of so much of my personal faith walk for several years. After much deliberation, Becky and I decided to return to Sedge Garden United Methodist Church in Kernersville where Becky was raised and where both we and our daughter were married. At a time when the mainstream Christian church is in such a state of decline, it was a hard decision. I had no significant issues with the theology coming from the pulpit of 1st Assembly. 1st Assembly was an early supporter of Motvation Ministry. I will forever be grateful for that support. The whole 1st Assembly experience was impactful. I have many old Quaker friends who cannot understand how I could find spiritual peace and motivation in such a conservative, evangelical church setting. My only answer is I found it hard to understand myself. While the outward manifestations of the faith are vastly different from those I experienced in the Quaker meetings of my young adulthood, the fundamental values I witnessed lived out in the body at 1st Assembly did not run counter to those beliefs. Without question, 1st Assembly was the most racially, economically, and demographically diverse church body I have ever participated in. Leaving that diversity was the hardest part of our decision to leave.

Since our return to SGUMC in 2015, Becky has become a mainstay in the traditional choral ministry of the church. She followed in her mother's footsteps and became a member of the church's Board of Trustees. I have taken a more reserved approach and avoided official responsibilities. Having lived through the split of the Winston-Salem Friends Meeting about which I wrote earlier, I have no desire to see any more of the underbelly of the church than necessary. I did teach a couple of Sunday School classes until COVID-19 shut down Sunday Schools for the duration. Once we returned to a regular Sunday School routine, I informed the classes I would not be available to continue that role. I never felt qualified to teach anybody anything in that environment. I used audio-video tools to bring other speakers and media into the classes. I didn't teach. Folks seemed to like it. I felt like a fraud.

Shortly before COVID-19's arrival, we welcomed a new pastor. Methodists tend to move their pastors on a regular schedule. Pastor Justin Lowe and family joined us as his first senior pastor placement. I should share this before I get too far into the weeds. As inferred earlier, I, by choice, had chosen not to become too involved in the life of the church. For some reason, Justin asked me to assume a leadership role for which I was woefully unqualified. He asked me to accept the role of

Lay Leader. I said no, and then said yes as he asked again and explained why he was asking. It was not a position I felt right about. But who was I to tell the new pastor 'No' again? Perhaps he had an insight, maybe a spiritual knowledge I could not tap. Accepting the role of Lay Leader meant I became a member (sometimes ex officio) on several central church committees-Pastor Parrish Church Relations, Budget & Finance, etc. It didn't take long to realize my placement was a big mistake.

The circumstances at SGUMC were different from the '60s, but there was still an underbelly of the church I did not want to be any part of. After a few short months "on the job" and participating in the committee sessions involving staffing issues, dealing with COVID-19 issues, and just overall new pastor-old line church member leadership, I resigned abruptly. I was already on a very thin rope in my faith walk. Being in the midst of that culture did not help. Becky and I still attend SGUMC. Becky loves her roles in the choir and the Trustees, and occasionally teaching in our Sunday School class. I don't feel much there. I am reminded of when I left the Quaker church many years ago. I remember sitting in a Sunday School class, the Koinonia Class, one Sunday morning.

Out of nowhere, I realized my experience had transformed from being one of spiritual growth and development to one of social justice and cultural activism. That was not what I was looking for in the church. I am not saying that is what I am experiencing at SGUMC. SGUMC has a lot going for it coming out of COVID. It is probably more engaged in the community's life and membership than any church I have attended other than WS First. I know whatever is not right with my relationship with God or the Church is no fault of the church on Sedge Garden Road. At least for now, we will continue to attend and be a part of that family, until the church (organization) does whatever it will do as an entity relating to the coming split over homosexuality. For now, I will continue to show up. I will continue a modest level of unofficial participation. We will see how God and I manage this ongoing time of encounter. I don't know what I think about God and His church these days. I'm pretty sure He is about as disillusioned with the modern-day church as I am. From this mere mortal's perspective, it is a painfully hard thing when something as foundational as the Christian church, on which so much of my faith has been walked through, finds itself in such jeopardy. A friend, John Bost, authored a book about this issue a few years ago. John wears many hats. I have been blessed to be present to hear him pray on numerous occasions and to read many of his mini-sermons in his Facebook posts. If ever there was such a thing, John is a "man of God." In his book <u>REPO: The Church in Foreclosure,</u> John draws from his experience as a realtor (just one of his many professional roles) to describe how the modern-day Christian church cannot possibly be what God, through Jesus, had in mind when the church was birthed. Perhaps all the discord and unrest in the church is part of the repossession process. Maybe God is reclaiming what is His. I am now 73 years old and will not be here to witness the resolution of this war. I pray my grandchildren might.

These past five years have been filled with taking several new and different paths. Since 2015 I have taken on two jobs, one part-time and on-ongoing, the other full-time off and on.

In 2015 I attended a job fair to go to work for RHINO Sports & Entertainment Services. RHINO is a Winston-Salem based company that provides support services for various sports, concerts, and other large public venues. One of my bucket list items was to find work in a minor-league professional baseball park on game days. My first job with RHINO in 2015 was to jump in a bucket truck and paint the big green wall in the outfield of the new minor league ballpark for the Winston-Salem DASH. That two-day assignment led to a several-week stint with the ground crew at the park. That brief stint was the only time I worked in the ballpark. It morphed into an ongoing licensed unarmed security spot through RHINO at Wake Forest University athletic events and some concerts and campus events requiring crowd management. I started in parking and was fortunate to be moved closer to the action. I work field-side for WFU football in the home team's tunnel to the field. I work courtside for basketball and am one of only 4-5 folks positioned to work near field-side at baseball.

The jobs pay little. It does pay something, and it gets me into the arena. Most days when I am "at work," I enjoy being in the arena. Then, all too often, that old demon rears its ugly head. I recognize that while I do get to engage with patrons in these environs (and I enjoy that), I don't belong in that world. It's embarrassing sometimes. Just before COVID, I worked at a huge Billy Joel concert at the WFU football stadium. It was a packed house. I was assisting with bag checks. The crowd was shoulder to shoulder coming through. Suddenly I heard a woman's voice call out, "Gene Gurley. Is that you, Gene Gurley?" I immediately knew somebody from my high school had spotted and recognized me after all these years. Indeed, it was two girl friends (not to be confused with girlfriends) from then. The crowd was moving along, so we couldn't talk. I did recognize her call and waved. I am certain the last place Pat ever expected to see Gene Gurley was working a bag check line at a Billy Joel concert. I was embarrassed. But it does pay a little, and after the fall of Motvation and the drawdown of such a portion of my retirement, even this little bit helps.

I need to be very clear here. Becky and I were never going to be wealthy. We never expected to be. Our career choices dictated that. We had been fortunate (in my case, after multiple tries) to get good educations and have jobs that made positive differences in people's lives. Even after I retired from Guilford and launched Motvation, we still were OK financially. I still understand how blessed I have been. I do appreciate the relative status of my situation. I can't get beyond my anger at having to lay down Motvation after investing the time and so much financial support. That is an ongoing conversation.

That said, RHINO has not been the only work opportunity to come my way. When I retired from Guilford, I was replaced by Paul Coscia, a staff member there for several years. Paul, also a Guilford alum, had been groomed in hopes he might take my job when I left. For whatever reasons, Paul left after two years. Paul landed on his feet as Director of Financial Aid at Salem College in Winston-Salem, a 250-year-old women's college founded by the Moravians, the early settlers of what would become Winston-Salem. Paul contacted me in 2017 and asked if I would help him for a few weeks while his front desk counselor was on maternity leave. I was available timewise and the money was helpful. So, I spent about ten weeks answering calls, managing walk-in traffic, and processing daily digital traffic between the office and government sources.

All in all, it was OK. It had been a long time since I had been solely responsible for much actual student traffic. By the time I retired from Guilford, I spent most of my time as a budget and personnel manager and liaison to other offices, faculty and staff, alums, donors, and Trustees. The job did fill the hours doing something constructive.

A couple of years later, Paul called again when Bekka, the staffer who had been away on maternal leave, decided she and her family were moving back up north, close to their families. I was to come and occupy the same position for a few weeks until the college decided what to do. Salem had been going through serious financial and accreditation difficulties. Like many small colleges, enrollment had been declining and fundraising was stagnant. I agreed again. This time I was there until the semester's end in the fall. At that time, Salem decided the position would not be staffed. With a significant decline in enrollment and related cash issues, Paul and his assistant Christy Chesnut would have to manage without a front desk staff.

Then, in June 2020, just after the presidential declaration of the COVID-19 pandemic in March, I got a call from Salem College. This time I was stunned. They wanted me to come in as Paul's replacement for 6-8 weeks. Paul was away on medical leave. Staff at Salem thought 6-8 weeks would cover Paul's remaining time needed to complete his medical treatment and return to work. I said I would be happy to help. After all, Paul had done a good job for me for several years. The least I could do was help him now. So, on Tuesday, July 6th, 2020, I began a full-time gig with different responsibilities, expecting to return to my routine and this writing project in six to eight weeks. I went to work assuming Paul would be back shortly after the start of classes in the fall. It serves no purpose to go into detail about how this saga evolved. Suffice it to say my original 6-8 commitment morphed into several extensions; first a few more weeks, then a couple more months. Paul was back at work mid-term.

Due to a variety of reasons, someone needed to help the financial aid office navigate through the maze. The flow of millions of dollars of federal and state COVID-19 relief funds, simultaneous with the arrival of a new college president with a massive new vision and mission for the college, required some assistance. I was that assistance. What was pitched as a 6–8-week fill-in while Paul was away became a nineteen-month stint, much of it working from home after students were sent home due to COVID. Finally, with new senior management on campus, and efforts underway to see real growth in enrollment, I told Paul and our new vice president I could not accept their invitation to continue beyond the start of the Spring 2022 semester. As the end date approached, I yielded again and extended it through the second week of February. That allowed me to close out all federal and state quarterly reports on COVID funding. I did sign one more short-term contract to complete and file the annual federal calendar year-end COVID funds report.

In 2019, while I was on staff at Salem for the second time, Becky and I took a wonderful ten-day road trip. We flew to Milwaukee to see the Cubs play the Brewers. We rented a car there and drove to Seattle to see the Mariners play the Padres. In between, we saw, up close and personal, a portion of this great land I had flown over occasionally but never seen from the ground. It was the trip of a lifetime, from the never-ending hay, corn, and wheat fields to the windmills to the magnificent road from Glacier National Park to Yellowstone. I pray that, as we get older, my mind remains intact to the point where I cannot remember sharing that time and space with the love of my life. That is a great fear. Genetically, my family tends to outlive their mental capacity. That was the kind of occasional retirement adventure I dreamed about. It was the kind of dream I have had to try to put away since Motvation.

With this last sojourn to Salem, I was able to again dream of doing something for our 50th wedding anniversary that would again offer a sharing of space and time in a beautiful setting. Late this past May and early June, a little less than one month before our anniversary Becky and I embarked on a thirteen-day road trip in Alaska. Rather than getting on a ship and sailing between ports, we decided to get in a car and drive. We flew to Anchorage on May 23rd, returning on June 5th, just before our anniversary on June 18th. Between May 23rd and June 5th, we drove south to Seward and Valdez and north as far as Fairbanks. We boarded two small boats for up-close viewing of wildlife and glaciers in the sounds. We took two small plane rides to land on and hike a glacier, and to visit the North Pole. A couple of weeks after returning, we enjoyed an anniversary celebration that Courtney (with some help from Scot) put together with a group of family and friends to help us share that memory and others accumulated over the fifty years. It was a good time. Time! Memories!

That sums it up. *On one level, I feel guilty for making those comparisons. On another level, I resent having to feel guilty.* The title of this chapter is ***"Does It Really Matter?"*** That turns out to be the ultimate question. Does it really matter? After all the stories, after all the memories, after all the successes and after all the failures- Does anything really matter? You know a good portion of my story- where I came from; what I did to earn a living most of my adult life. You know something about what I try to access or do to find joy and pleasure (happiness??) in life. You know my most significant life experience was having Becky Smith enter my life and say yes to me. I would forsake everything else this world has presented or could ever offer to me to be able to walk this road with her again, trying to undo what I should have never done, trying to fix what I messed up.

I am getting old, and I know that is how it is. I have been blessed with good health. I can still outwalk and outwork most men my age. My mind is still clear and agile enough to hold my own. I worry about that. My daddy and brother both had major heart attacks by the time they were in their late 60s. Becky has seen to it that I have eaten healthier than they did in their time in eastern North Carolina. My brother had a debilitating stroke when he was eighty. He never fully recovered. For two years, until his death, he could not speak with any clarity. He required assistance to eat. He would cry at the drop of a hat. Buddy and Katy had been happily married since he returned from the Korean War. I know Buddy would have given anything to be able to hug his love one more time. Katy was there with him every day through it all.

I suspect it is pretty normal for men, women too perhaps, to reflect at this station of life, to reflect on *their* lives. The problem I have now, having reached this point, is I want to know- **Does it really matter?** Does any of this really matter at all? Perhaps I got it all wrong a long time ago. Perhaps my struggle to feel happy, to enjoy the moment without the almost constant fear of failure or defeat, to know in my bones that I have value, that I am loved without reservation- perhaps it should not have been so hard to be that person. I'll never know. There is so much *"this me"* will never experience or never experience again. And *this me* resents that fact. Moreover, *this me* resents that the events of my times and events of my life were lived with such a pervasive and ever-present shadow that even those good times and peak moments could never be thoroughly enjoyed, shared, or appreciated- not to the level they had the potential to be enjoyed, shared, appreciated.

When Becky and I visit our daughter and her family in Mississippi, sometimes we fly; sometimes we drive. It depends on the schedule, the need to take or bring back baggage, or our desire to take a side trip on either end of the main journey. One thing is always certain though. It is a long drive. Sometimes we break it up and spend the night on the west side of Atlanta before going the rest of the way.

Another thing is inevitable on the return drive. We are almost home, seemingly just minutes away, when we approach the exit from I-85 to get onto the NC Hwy 52 North to Winston-Salem. I get the sense that is where I am now in this exercise-almost home.

No matter how much we enjoy our visits to MS, it is good to get home. Somehow, this old farmhouse on top of this hill in Kernersville has become my refuge. I don't know if that is a good thing. It is easy to hide in a refuge. It can take real effort and motivation to leave a refuge. If nothing really matters, why work so hard to escape it?

I feel like I have reached the off-ramp to NC Hwy 52 North and am close to the driveway I so long to enter. When I see that front porch and Becky's car, I know I'm home. When I walk in the door and am greeted by my best little friend, I know I am where I am supposed to be.

I cannot count the hours I have labored over these pages. As I have read and re-read my recollections recorded in these pages, I have come to realize there is so much more I need to say, so much more I need to 'get out' of my system. I want to understand what that means insofar as addressing my initial mission here. If nothing really matters, then why bother doing anything? But, what if? Oh- that again! What if somewhere in the bowels of all that undigested biomass, there is a something that might matter- if not to anyone else, to me? Is it worth taking another deeper dive into all this history, just for my own satisfaction? Or am I just forestalling a decision that beckoned the questions raised in these pages? Can I really give up on the question if there is any chance that something does matter, that somehow, I might be able to take control and alter the pace of time relative to life's moments? Is the potential of that morsel sufficient to endure the continuing search, given the costs recited herein? I don't know! Is it worth a try?

Chapter 20

I'M STILL TIRED!!

WELL- HERE WE are. When I set out on this exercise, I had no idea how difficult it would be. Writing *The Letter* seemingly rolled off the keyboard. It was almost like it had written itself and was waiting for the rest of me to catch up. I thought what came next would flow as easily. It did not. Some of that was because I have never kept a journal and have never maintained calendars of my activities beyond the time surrounding those events. Therefore, I had to recall from memory people, places, events, and stories relevant to the task. I discovered there was way too much content for the pages. I constantly found myself deviating from my mission. I stated in *The Letter* what I wanted to do at the conclusion of my letter. I believe I was clear in *The Letter* about where I was at the start of this review. I had a decision to make. I wanted to take inventory of the peaks and valleys, the good and bad days, from various angles and decide.

Once I embarked on a mental journey through the years, it became uncomfortable on the one hand and painfully all-consuming on the other. I found myself constantly shifting from becoming totally engaged in recalling an event or a relationship to struggling to remember timelines and sequences of events. I found myself getting sucked into memories of good times that I wanted to go on and on. Then, when I came upon a time or event I wanted to pretend or wish never happened, I found myself up against a wall. The words would not come. Just like in the real time of life, I found myself shrinking from what I knew I should be doing. I made excuses about what else I needed to work on. One of the most damning discoveries when I was about two-thirds of the way through was the realization I had avoided, or relegated to only a brief mention, certain people or events that warranted far more attention. Whether for good or for bad, these people and events formed the fabric of the story and are inextricably meshed with the story. They warranted more attention and follow-up than the brief one or two comments in their initial mentions, or worse, their total absence from mentioning. I don't know whether these brief mentions or absolute disappearance from subsequent conversations was intentional or simply the failure of an inexperienced writer to follow a thread. This was never about the writing. It was always about me trying to make an informed, well-disciplined decision, based on a thorough and objective review of the peaks and valleys of the journey and the story they tell.

So, when I got to that point, I had to look for windows where I should have paused and reflected upon the ongoing role of that person or event on the continuously evolving thread. The problem then became how to do that without getting bogged down in the process. That is of no concern to me now. My original letter was straightforward. The sole purpose of what followed was to guide the decision-making. There are family and friends who I love dearly. Specifically, there are now grown children and grandchildren who I want to know all of Pappy in a way they would otherwise never know him. They have that right.

One thing I have discovered during this adventure, mainly because of my exposure to and friendship with my Christian brothers in the New Canaan Society, is my story is not so unique. Sure, the particulars of people, places, and events are mine. But, the life of successes, failures, accomplishments, and disappointments that is my life is not unique. We all experience these combinations of life's moments in one way or another. So, as noted previously, this review and assessment process has been taxing, both therapeutic and cathartic. It has been revealing. The overarching dilemma concerning the peaks and valleys, the successes and the failures, is universal. Everyone encounters both in varying degrees of intensity and duration and must live with the consequences of both, at least until they make a choice otherwise.

I do not wish to spend any more time on this exercise. I am still very tired; if anything, more so. Nothing in this exercise has quenched that fatigue. But, somehow, something is just not quite right. That whole "what if" thing, just won't go away. I am tired; but curious.

In Act 3, Scene 1 of William Shakespeare's tragedy, "*Hamlet*," Hamlet speaks.

"To be, or not to be, that is the question:
Whether 'tis nobler in the mind to suffer
The slings and arrows of outrageous fortune,
Or to take arms against a sea of troubles
And by opposing end them. To die—to sleep,"

[From the Second Quarto of Hamlet (1604)]

"To be or not to be." To live or not to live. That is indeed the question. It turns out I am not breaking new ground here. This question of whether this mortal journey, and all its encounters and experiences, is worth the cost, is a question that has captured the minds of critical thinkers since recorded history began, maybe before that. I didn't ask for this. Either my (or your) existence materialized here as a matter of simple cosmic evolution in a micro sense. Or were we placed here, within this moment in time, by a Power we call God? I have tried hard to get my mind around all this.

What can my presence (or lack of) on this little speck mean to any Creator? That is a question apart from what my presence really means to others with whom I am sharing this ride- either in the moment or over some period as time moves on. I am familiar with the Christian Biblical view on the answer to that question. I want to believe. In a macro sense, I want to believe life has some universal value and meaning. I want to believe I have some meaningful purpose. I want to believe a Creator (God) is at work. I believe no matter how convoluted any moment in time is, there is value in participating in those moments. I want to believe the value is worth the cost.

Epilogue

The Letter– A Postscript

*IT SEEMS LIKE forever since I wrote **The Letter**, raising the issue of the dilemma I was facing and wrestling with for a long time. After hundreds of hours of reminiscing and reflecting, I am still unsure what all this means and what I am supposed to do now. Somehow, the situation seems to fit. Most of my life has been filled with moments of indecision and prevarication. Why should now be any different? That said– I believe NOW may be different.*

Cutting through all the rhetoric and reflecting, I realize that through it all, I am blessed to have two anchors that will always keep me from venturing too far into unknown waters: my faith walk and my family. I cannot give up on the journey I have stumbled along since my teen years. While I cannot articulate any understanding of the deep, miraculous, and steadfastness of that Presence, I know I cannot forsake its reality. Secondly, I could never willingly do anything to cause pain to Becky or my children (and now, grandchildren.) I love them too much ever to go there. And, I know they love me likewise. I think I have sensed the presence of both of these anchors all along. Earlier, I commented that my struggles with these issues are in no way unique to me, and by comparison, my challenges, disappointments, and failures are not noteworthy. Therein lies the epiphany of this entire exercise. My story is my story. It is not yours. My successes, *challenges, disappointments, and failures are mine and mine alone. You have your successes, challenges, disappointments, and failures. My anchors are mine and I now know they are strong enough to withstand any force that would seek to separate me from them. **My challenge to anyone who reads this epistle is this: Find-Your-Anchors!** They are there. They may not be the same as mine. But they are there. **Find them, latch onto them, and do not ever let go!***

Relative to my faith walk, I said earlier I do want to believe. Having solidified that want, I must live accordingly. I don't see how I can avow a desire to live in a relationship with the Presence and willingly walk toward The Darkness. I don't know how getting up each morning and putting that commitment into action will take shape. I have no illusion that the internal struggle between the peaks and valleys and the successes and failures will suddenly disappear. I'm not that naïve.

Despite all the failures and disappointments, and moments of utter self-hate, I now know my life has been incredibly blessed in the ways that matter. This late in the story, nothing is going to change in any significant way materially. I must learn to accept that and live accordingly. I have come to believe that my existence has been of value; I have had a meaningfully positive influence on others; in ways and degrees I can never know. For that recently acquired understanding, I am grateful. I also must accept that I will not achieve any of those ambitions and dreams I fantasized about when I was younger- not going to happen. Now, I am grateful it is not too late to bask in the glory of what I do have. I have been blessed to live a life since my early twenties with a marvelous partner. I understood that from the beginning. I have tried to show her just how aware of that blessing I am. What I have not done, and now must do, is consciously and intentionally remind myself of that fact every day, particularly when those tugs and nudges from the dark places try to take control of the narrative. Together our lives have been immeasurably enriched by two children, and now three grandchildren. Neither child ever caused me one minute of stress. I've never lost trust in them. I have always known they love me. Much of my distress leading to this exercise relates to my sense of failure relative to their upbringing. They turned out great. I still feel like I was not always there when I should have been. I cannot undo that now. All I can do is be there now for them and the grandkids. I cannot be absent from that responsibility, and that opportunity.

I have written much about the challenge of Time; how Time seems to be a fleeting, ethereal presence when the occasion evokes happiness and joy. Then, when the moment, or occasion, is a result of, or a trigger to, a valley, a failure, a disappointment, or a shortcoming, then it seems to linger, to hover, to settle in for the duration. Not only does it seem to vary its pace, depending on the direction of the sensory experience, it also seems to pick and choose when to return to the scene and resurrect its emotional stimulus. I can no longer allow Time to be in charge. The fact is Time is a constant. It doesn't actually change pace or cycle. That is all my mental and emotional construct. I must intentionally seek mental and emotional support from resources I believe align with the God I just said I want to pursue a closer living relationship with.

Finally, I cannot do anything but try to be as good a husband, father, grandfather, and friend as possible. I am reminded of the scriptural reference I cited when we launched Motvation Ministry. We used these verses as the guiding thought for all we attempted to do with the students we reached out to.

Philippians 4:8-9 *"8 Finally, brothers and sisters, whatever is true, whatever is noble, whatever is right, whatever is pure, whatever is lovely, whatever is admirable—if anything is excellent or praiseworthy—think about such things. 9 Whatever you have learned or received or heard from me, or seen in me—put it into practice. And the God of peace will be with you." NIV Version*

My challenge is to be a better student of this message than I have been up to now. There is still time to make this transformation. Now, more than ever, I want to believe the value is worth the cost! I want to grow old(er) with my sweetheart. I want to be present when Scot or Courtney need me to be present as they approach their mid-life years. I want to share in Abby's, Owen's, and Julia's ascents to adulthood and all that implies. I want to help them learn from my story, using Phil. 4:8,9 as my daily guide. I must be willing to absorb the cost.

05/05/2023

ABOUT THE AUTHOR

ANTHONY GURLEY is not famous. He is not a celebrity, athlete, politician, or business tycoon. His is not a household name. He is just an ordinary guy with a story to tell, one told under the umbrella of asking a bigger question about life relating to daily successes and victories, and failures and disappointments, both personal and professional.

Anthony grew up in public housing in eastern North Carolina in the 1950s and 60s, the youngest of five children, six years younger than his closest sibling. His father walked out on him and the family at home just as he turned twelve.

A stellar student and leader in high school, graduating in 1967, Anthony spent the next ten years earning a four-year degree at Guilford College, taking time away on two occasions working, getting married, and starting a family. He spent thirty years at his alma mater as the Director of Financial Aid, retiring in 2009 to launch Mo-T-Vation Ministry, providing scholarships and mentors to college-going Christian artists and athletes.

Through the years, Anthony has battled the rigors of poor self-image and lack of self-esteem. His daddy's words to him as a child, "*Get out of the way. I can't see through muddy water,*" and "*Don't ask me for a damn thing,*" have haunted him in his struggle to value his own self-worth. Through it all, he has been blessed with his wife, Becky, for fifty-one years, two children, and three grandchildren. He also acknowledges awareness of a faith walk which has always been at the core of his journey, even when he was not in step with The One leading the way.

In *Deadly Dilemma*, Anthony unsparingly opens wide the doors to his journey in the hope that others might find a path to confronting their struggles and their failures, and in the process, discover their life-saving answers to that bigger question. *Are those moments of victory and success, happiness and joy, and peaks of cherishable memories sufficient in number, scope, magnitude, and frequency to outweigh the valleys of failure, disappointments, fear, and isolation, that often color the landscape of life?*

www.anthonygurley.com
anthony@anthonygurley.com

Printed in the USA
CPSIA information can be obtained
at www.ICGtesting.com
LVHW021454280124
769814LV00072B/2207